iF i CAN'T BE DEAD, HoW CAN i LiVE?

Dealing With Feeling In Recovery

All stories are true. All names have been changed.
The author is grateful to the women who had the courage
to tell their stories. For some, it meant healing old wounds.

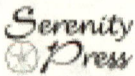

Copyright © 2002 by Martha Crikelair Wohlford
Published by Serenity Press

All rights reserved.
No part of this book may be reproduced, stored in a retrieval system,
or transmitted by any means, electronic, mechanical, photocopying,
recording, or otherwise, without written permission from the author.

ISBN 13: 978-0-9787981-2-3
ISBN 10: 0-9787981-2-0

Cover Design: Martha Wohlford

Printed in the U.S.A.
Printed March 2009

About the Book

This is a book written from the heart to touch the heart.

The purpose is to give support and hope to women in recovery, to dispel the fear of treatment, and to show how to deal with feelings without drinking or using drugs in everyday life situations.

While the book primarily focuses on women, it is a helpful tool for anyone living a 12-Step program.

It is a journey of recovery from awareness of the problem, through treatment and life after treatment. Anyone who thinks alcohol may be a problem in their life will identify with the women who share their stories, their innermost thoughts and feelings.

Most important, the book gives suggestions for dealing with everyday situations as a sober, healthy person.

The theme is simple: I can't, He can, I think I'll let Him.

In the course of writing the book, the manuscript was shared with several women in recovery and with a close friend who thought she might have a problem with alcohol but who was too frightened to go to A.A. Reading the first 60 pages gave her the courage to go to her first A.A. meeting and she's been sober ever since. So, before even going to press, the book was a success!

Dedicated to all the

courageous women who made it possible.

You know who you are.

Those in need will appreciate your service.

Thank you!

Table of Contents

Pre-Recovery 1
   Awareness 3
   Treatment...11
The First Year 47
Living One Day At a Time in AA 50
   Still Sober 53
Divorce 56
   When All is Lost in the Process..............................62
   Affirmations..67
   Suggestions for going through divorce 68
Children 69
   Cunning, Baffling, Powerful – and Patient 73
   The Daughter's Point of View 78
   Suggestions for helping your children 80
Death..82
   A Love Story 84
   A Child's Suicide 96
   Suggestions for dealing with death 102
Health/Injury/Hospitalization 104
   Gaining on Pain – A Delicate Balance 109
   When Nothing Seems to Work 111
   Still a 'Pickle' 113
   Suggestions for health problems 114
Relationships 116
   Suggestions for relationships 125
Career/Finances 127
   All You Have to do is Dream 129
   A Wrong Way and A Right Way 131
   Suggestions for career and finances 133
God Stories 134
   The Signs Were Everywhere! 139

  Ask, and you shall Receive 141
  A Wheel of Fortune 143
  Suggestions for recognizing God 145
Getting Professional Help 146
  Suggestions for getting professional help 159
Other Issues 161
  National Tragedy 9/11/01 161
  Using the Internet 164
  News Media 166
About the Author 170

Pre-Recovery

Alone in her family. Depressed. Afraid of hurting her children. Hating herself. Hating her husband. Hopeless. Helpless. A black hole so large she could see no light. Despair. Unable to get in touch with any positive emotion. Planning her suicide.

That's where Angie's story begins.

Having a small life insurance policy was the basis for months of obsessing on how to relieve herself of the overwhelming despair engulfing her while keeping up the front of wife, mother, businesswoman. She still had enough pride and sense of who she once was to know that shooting herself was not an option. Too messy. Too much for the kids to deal with. Something that would haunt them forever, she said. We were sitting in a park on a wooden bench. She shook her head and hunched over, elbows on her knees, head down, her hands cupping her chin. We watched in silence as the squirrels chased each other. Kids swung on swings with mothers watching their every move. I waited for Angie to continue.

She confided that in the bottom of her basket of hopelessness, she knew there was the realization that she could hurt the hell out of her husband, but not her babies...her precious children who meant everything to her and whom she was destroying with her disease.

"I didn't know I had a fatal disease," she said. "I thought I was insane. I was crazy. I was desperate. But sick? That concept was unfamiliar. I only knew I was consumed with guilt."

So, how would she deal with the monster within who wanted her dead?

She told me it had to look like an accident. She could even envision the headline "Mother of Two Killed as Sports Car Hits Interstate Overpass."

Her ironic smile contrasted with the tears welling up in her eyes, which teetered on her lower lids before tumbling down her cheeks. She wiped them away with her sleeve.

"I obsessed about this," she said. "I figured every angle. Then the night I was ready, after several drinks for courage and authenticity and another argument with my husband, I climbed into my little sports convertible, turned the key, and gunned the engine. I shifted into gear, mentally contemplating the process and envisioning the result. And then someone drove into my driveway and I had no way out." She stared ahead, the eyes now like steel, her jaw set.

She shook her head.

"I have little recollection of my anger, of calling an old-time friend a bastard," she said. "I thought, how could you do this to me...don't you know I'm going to kill myself? I wanted him out of my way. I can remember running toward him as he got out of his car, flailing my arms. I hit him repeatedly, then broke down sobbing uncontrollably."

A few moments went by, then she said, "I couldn't even kill myself properly."

Awareness

That was the beginning of Angie's journey. She doesn't know when she became an alcoholic, but recalls that when she was 22 years old she was aware she might have a problem with alcohol and feared she would one day have to deal with it. But at that time in her life, she boasted she "could drink a date under the table and drive him home, thank you."

It was not easy for her to recount her story after so many healthy years. She said it was like recalling a bad dream that at one time haunted her, followed her, reminded her of how she once hated herself. But knowing Angie as she is today, I convinced her that it was important to tell her story. We met a few days later at the same park, where she reluctantly began remembering her past.

"I began drinking on my 18th birthday, the day I also began smoking. Swim team obligations went out the window at that point. Besides, the younger swimmers were beating me at every meet. My National Honor Society status would have been impossible to obtain if I hadn't received it my junior year. I just floated through that last semester of high school, doing as little as possible. It was like I was another person," she said, noting that her parents had expressed concern over her grades and her newfound weekend social life.

"Drinking let me break out as the oldest in a strict Catholic family. After graduation, I went to a large university where I became a member of the sailing team as a freshman – and you know how sailors drink," she smiled, recalling the "fun" times, traveling around the country to other schools, successfully competing and having a great time.

"We partied so much my freshman year that when I returned for my sophomore year no one on the racing team had a high enough grade point to be an officer of the sailing club, and the university disbanded the organization until we could get our grades up," she shook her head, a slight grin on her face, then continued. "Of course, I left mid-year with an 'I'll show them' attitude and ended up at the strict Catholic women's college where my parents had originally wanted me to go."

She chuckled, recalling how her drinking was sorely hampered by nuns who would try to smell her breath as she shakily wrote her name in the sign-in book at the end of every evening out.

"Somehow I managed to cope, always looking for the next party, planning outrageous ways to have fun while getting away with breaking every rule of the school." With a lot of work, she was able to balance her fun times drinking with maintaining her studies, allowing her to graduate with a respectable grade point.

"It's almost comical how alcoholics can juggle their lives to survive," she said. "But that only lasts so long."

She began her career as a journalist back in the small home town she had once escaped, living in the home she grew up in with the same five younger siblings.

"Talk about cramping my style! But, as a successful budding alcoholic, I managed to find a guy who drank like I did and, needless to say, honorably escaped the house following a huge wedding to my drinking buddy where all the 'right' people attended the country club reception."

In the months prior to the wedding, she knows she worried her mother.

"Mom would stay up late waiting for us," she said. "The greeting became routine: 'Are you drunk again?' If my fiance was in the same shape, she would often call a taxi rather than let him drive the 20 minutes to his home."

This was decades before the slogan "Friends don't let friends drive drunk," when people routinely drove drunk with little consequence.

Angie said her mother was always there for her, a kindred soul who blazed her own trail in difficult times, who could leave a drink half-finished because she'd had enough or just didn't want it.

"Many of those half-emptied glasses were finished by me or my siblings over the years of my parents' entertaining in the family home."

Following the wedding, she and her new husband conveniently moved to another part of the country where family could not monitor their drinking. They each chose more exciting work and got on with life, which meant buying a sailboat and cruising the Bahamas (with plenty of beer stowed and money for good rum).

"Everything we did involved drinking," she said, "and everyone we associated with drank like we did. It was the best of times, even though we scrimped and saved for the next bottle, choosing to eat peanut butter sandwiches so we could have our booze...even if it was only one bottle for the week when times were really tough. I didn't dare let my parents know how I was living. I was already experiencing the shame and consequences of my lifestyle, which meant covering up or avoiding the truth."

The reality was that they were able to work, to function, while continuing to drink. She said that one bottle a week eventually increased to a bottle a night.

"My hangovers were always horrendous, but I always figured it would be different tomorrow," she said. "My husband's work eventually led to his being gone weeks at a time as either crew or captain on charter yachts. It was then that I began to drink alone."

They eventually had two children, a boy and a girl. Angie said God must have been watching over her, because alcohol did not appeal to her during pregnancy.

"Coming out of the delivery room following natural childbirth of my second child, my daughter, I wanted a beer and a roast beef sandwich. I was ready to get on with the old life right away. Years later I realized that I had lost 24 hours in the birth of my son four years before. I thought he was born on a Thursday, but it was a day later, after I was given the option of either being given more drugs or having my baby. I chose to have my baby rather than have drugs further delay labor. I was addicted then but didn't know it."

Angie continued as a functioning, productive member of society, not only with her own business, which she began "before they burned the bra," but an exciting air charter business with her husband.

"On the outside, we were the successful family – nice home in an upscale neighborhood, two cars, a dog, private school for the kids," she smiled. "We looked just great on the outside."

Five o'clock became synonymous with the first drink.

"If my husband wasn't home, I started without him, never letting anyone know, ever, how much I drank. I controlled my drinking when I saw clients and made sure I looked good and didn't reek of alcohol. But then, how could I make an honest evaluation of how others saw me? Denial created a facade of success and happiness. Putting on the mask became as essential as my underwear," she said.

Behind closed doors, a stealthy killer lurked, waiting patiently as the years of drinking accumulated. Angie went from making sure her husband had his rum and Coke ready as soon as he walked in the door to cuddling her gallon of Gallo before bedtime.

"It took years, but it was *so* fast when I turned the corner," she recounted. "I went from wanting a drink to needing a drink. Alcohol, the friend that helped me be funny and acceptable, became my enemy. I was at war with not wanting to drink and having to drink...not during the day, though. To drink in the morning after hanging over the toilet bowl to appease my splitting head would have meant I was REALLY an alcoholic. That's why I waited until 5 o'clock...I thought everybody drinks at that time so why be any different from the next guy?"

But she knew she was.

When bedtime stories turned to waking the children at three o'clock in the morning to clean their rooms, when the fear of hitting them without wanting to instilled a gut-wrenching fear, when morning business appointments had to be moved to the afternoon so she could pull herself together, when she made commitments to clients in the evening that she couldn't recall the next morning – the signs of destruction were everywhere, yet Angie could not stop drinking.

"I continued not because I wanted to, but because it was survival," she said. I would have a drink before bedtime to relieve my nerves, to kick start a fitful sleep...a few before going to a friend's house to make sure I'd have my share and could be sociable, and, of course, a few when I got home because I still hadn't had enough."

She was told later on that normal people don't think that way or do those things. Toward the end, everything revolved around planning her drinking to still be functional and putting up the front that becomes the nightmare of every alcoholic.

"I thought, my God, how can I keep this up? I was exhausted living the lie," she said.

Then total chaos arrived – not welcomed but unavoidable. Her live-in housekeeper, the only bit of sanity and stability within her home, left. The glamorous business she had with her husband took a turn for the worse, with overwhelming lease payments and payroll. The children required more and more attention because she no longer had help. Then, the final blow. Her father, who had struggled with cancer for almost two years, was dying. No amount of beer, wine or booze could solve the problems.

"I found myself back and forth across the country to try to help with my father, but I was more of a hindrance," she said. "Two weeks before he died, the ultimate 'check' on the list of questions to determine if I was alcoholic occurred. I lost several hours, blacked out in my parents' home in the presence of my siblings, with everyone thinking they'd have to bury me before my father."

But God works in strange ways.

"Early on, my dad was a good drinking buddy of mine. He'd arrive with fine French wines that we would savor for the first sip or two, then slug down to open yet another bottle. It drove my mother crazy. She couldn't understand why he would make such a big deal about bringing wine to my house, but we both knew why. He was allergic to something in gin, so in the early days, when we still lived in the area where I grew up, he would come visit our little apartment and drink his martinis. We never cared that he sneezed his head off."

But the blackout was downright frightening. She said that in the past she could remember and account for most of her actions, no matter how much booze she had consumed. This time she had no recollection of those hours.

"Zip. Gone. Forever," she said, snapping her fingers and shaking her head. "Next came the predictable guilt and shame, the promises of change, the admission of my problem. But I still had denial in the back of my brain. It was meeting with my father that changed everything. There was no longer an escape."

Behind the closed door, he looked at her in a way that was different.

"I know now that it was how one alcoholic can look at another and know their whole life history of pain and despair. He talked to me gently one-on-one and somehow got the promise from me that I would go to treatment," she said. "He knew I would not go to AA on my own."

She would tell herself, Sure, Dad, anything you ask of me...maybe if I do what you ask you won't die...maybe that's the answer. Maybe it's all my fault and we can fix it quick. That was the last time she was able to talk with him.

On Sept. 14, 1979, Angie's father died. He saved enough awareness in his comatose state to wait for her and squeeze her hand, confirmation that the six children were finally together for their mother.

"After the heart-wrenching funeral attended by many people, I returned home to my life, grieving his loss and burdened with the promise I had made to him," she said. "I was angry at him for dying and extracting the promise for me to go to treatment. The commitment now hung over my head like a dead albatross, and with every drink I took from that point on, I knew I was betraying him, delaying my commitment."

Angie said the end of her drinking came so quickly she hardly remembers all the events leading up to the constant thoughts of suicide. She made the appointment for treatment "just in case," and, functional alcoholic that she was, worked feverishly so "they'd have money coming in while I'm gone, thank you!"

With suicide foiled, battered and bruised from the fight, she packed her bags and boarded the plane as scheduled, to a treatment center far away from home, across the country.

"I know it's stupid now, but I was really concerned about what friends and neighbors would think if I were to seek help," she said. "I just told everyone I was going to help my mother for a while."

Treatment – October 1979

As a good alcoholic, Angie had put certain "conditions" on her promise. Her father had already chosen where he wanted her to go for treatment, one of the top facilities in the country. In filling out her requests on the application to the center, she specified "private room." She arrived with her typewriter and guitar.

"Obviously, I had no concept of 'treatment,' what 'detox' was or anything else relating to recovery," she said. "I didn't even know I was suffering from a disease. Crazy was good enough – an acceptable, believable diagnosis. Only people out of their mind would want to take their own life, right?"

Angie has only vague recollections of arriving at the treatment center.

"I know that the plane taking me had a layover in a big city before going on to my destination, and I am also aware that my husband and others at home were worried I would get off the plane and take some sort of devious detour more to my liking, avoiding the arrival at my destination," she said. "I also remember that I refused to have a drink on the plane. The last drink I had was October 23, 1979, at a restaurant specializing in barbecue ribs. It was a vodka and tonic with lime. I had only two of them and then dinner. If I had ordered another it would have meant I REALLY DID have a problem, so to prove to my husband and friend (the one who stopped my suicide in the driveway and who had been to the same treatment center two years prior) that I could still control it, I purposely, pointedly and pathetically, stopped at two. I remember thinking the day I arrived at treatment that it was the day before my sister's birthday, October 25. If I had not made this mental association, I probably would not have remembered the exact date of my sobriety without searching my personal records later on."

As Angie got off the plane, someone approached her, called her by name, helped her retrieve her luggage and then put her in a station wagon for the hour drive to the treatment center.

"The driver kept asking if I wanted to stop for one last drink," she said. "I told him no, although my anxiety level was incredible and I'm sure a drink would have calmed my nerves."

As they drove into the tree-lined road leading to the center, Angie recounts having a strange feeling of peace, that maybe this beautiful place could help her.

"Just as I was appreciating the surroundings, I turned negative, probably out of fear," she said. "My anger flared. I became frustrated, thinking once again that it would be better to be dead than where I was. I dug my heels in and allowed my attitude to take over, but like any other alcoholic, I also knew I would have to do a lot of conning to get my way."

The Admitting Department put her through the usual hospital-type intake process and she remembers commenting on wanting a private room.

"They just smiled at me as if saying 'poor dear,'" she said. "That also irritated me. Then they went through all my things, even taking my aspirin, and put me in a small room for detox, which I was to experience for the first time."

A smallish woman probably in her 50s with graying hair and glasses walked in and said, "So, I understand you want to kill yourself."

"I remember being extremely negative and nasty to her, challenging where she got her information. Obviously, someone had 'ratted.' She probably could tell what I was feeling just by looking at me." Angie was given Librium to bring her temperature and blood pressure to normal and fructose, "the dentist's answer for a hangover."

"I remember being sick to my stomach," she continued. "They provided relaxation tapes and soothing music and someone came often to check on me. I have little recollection of those first two days of detox, but remember mentally and physically struggling over what was happening to me. Anything I am recalling now could easily be challenged by someone who REALLY knows what went on, so I'll begin where I have a written log knowledge of treatment. One of the questions I asked that impish woman after detox has lingered throughout my sobriety: If I can't be dead, how can I live?"

The feeling of total aloneness and bitterness against people you know really mean well...the frustration...
Angie's journal October 26

On October 26th Angie was transferred to her unit. She met her roommate, Maggie, who immediately became a target of resentment because she did not get the private room she had ordered.

"Maggie was about 10 years older than I and a nurse, and I couldn't for the life of me understand how anyone could have such a fabulous sense of humor in such a horrible situation. Surely I HAD landed in a nut house!"

Maggie was also a non-smoker, and Angie soon discovered they were the only two on the entire unit who didn't smoke.

"I was dumfounded how anyone could see anything laughable in the given situation, but I know now that God sure works in strange ways. This woman was pretty wacky but had a heart of gold and was a perfect match for me," she said. "Her jokes helped me keep things light, but I still had dismal thoughts and plenty of anger."

I have no urge for phone calls from home or a desire to write or be written to. It's like "ok, I'm here. Now stow it and survive any damn way you want to...with or without me."
Angie's journal October 26

Their room overlooked a lake and Angie wrote in her journal about wanting to get some good black and white photos. It had snowed before she arrived and she wanted to show her children what snow looked like. Having grown up in Florida, neither had yet seen snow.

At this point they are so very far away, as is everything else. I wonder if I'll get to the point of wanting to return. I still am not convinced I want to get well, although I am coming to grips with the thought that, like everyone here, I have a problem that is going to get worse. I am torn between love and hate for my husband and hope to hell he does not call, particularly if there is more bad news. I resent seeing our friend's name as a referral on all the goddamn forms I have to fill out...
Angie's journal October 26

On October 27, following a long counseling session, Angie took a walk in the woods outside her unit.

"I was feeling less helpless with the knowledge of what had happened to me. After two days of testing I was told I actually had a brain left," she smiled. The psychologists told her she had not done any mental damage to herself – yet!

"I logged in my journal that I had 'whipped through'

the tests like I do everything else," she said. "I was pretty arrogant, but I was no better than anyone else. I was hurting like everyone else, and needed help like everyone else, yet there was a smug superiority in my journal entries, probably masking my insecurity at the time."

I collected dandelions, maple leaves turned a golden brown, milkweed about to burst, spreading its silken seed pods for next year's harvest. The goldenrod, so prevalent in Wisconsin only a month and a half ago, is beginning to turn its winter dead brown, though there were a few sprigs to add color to a fall bouquet. Some things I have not been able to identify – weeds with nut-like nodules, fuzzy balls of varying sizes combined with the tired green of fall and the brown of beginning winter. The beauty of the lake with the evergreens, the distant homes overlooking this place, remind me of the days of my childhood when the lake near home was about to give up its fluid gray to the white harshness of winter ice. The trees now in limbo are in such contrast to the lushness of palm trees back home. The grass is still green, peppered with leaves that have now lost their reddish and yellowish hue for the brown that signifies the final coming of winter and the giving up of fall.

Angie's journal October 27

Although Angie was not totally aware of the transition, her thinking and emotions began to change. She said she expressed amazement that after only a few short days she had the urge to write, to record the beauty around her even though stark. Something was happening.

"Deep down, I knew I would again write some poetry, maybe a song. I remember being elated over the thought that I could possibly do these things again."

She spoke with her four-year-old daughter that day, assuring her that mommy was okay, "up north" for a while, but that she'd be coming home soon.

"I still had resentment against my husband," she said. "But that night, I got out my guitar for the first time in many years, strung it with new strings, and held it like a forgotten child. As my drinking progressed, I had stopped playing. This fact, and the realization that I was six months behind reading my *National Geographic* magazines – something I did faithfully for many years prior to and every month since recovery – was also evidence that I had a problem."

After nine years of classical piano training, Angie took up the guitar at age 18, just when Joan Baez began her career. Throughout college, she said her guitar went everywhere with her.

"I sang in folk groups, with individuals and also on my own – on and off campus, in coffee shops, bars and anywhere I was welcome," she said. "It was great fun. But looking back, I remember a night when I had too much to drink and my fingers wouldn't work. I had to put the guitar down and continue singing with my two partners, who could still pluck away. This happened again and again...I didn't know when to stop drinking. I also remember my friends being upset with me."

At the treatment center, her guitar brought her back to the old, good times.

"I needed to play as much as my 'inmates,' wanted to hear. Music was such a welcome release from the intense routine of the day."

They decided *Bottle of Wine* would be a good theme song for their unit...*when ya gonna let me get sober...*

I think of my dad, especially walking in the woods and

knowing that he is here with me, encouraging me, happy that I will overcome. I look at this vase of fall beauty and think of the farm, of the poplar trees whistling in the breeze, the blackberry bushes now barren, only steps from dad's grave, of how the cemetery road must be similar to the pine-tree path I just left while picking my collections. Perhaps it is significant that I am here, where it is so similar to the farm. Sun-and-Fun Florida is so far away. My world of reality, where I learned early to appreciate the seasons in the north, may be my solace these next few weeks.
Angie's journal October 27

Angie feels that particular Sunday marked the beginning of her acceptance.

"Looking back after many years of recovery I know that acceptance took place long before I recognized it or I wouldn't have gone for help," she said. "Reading literature on alcoholism made me look at the previous six months as happening for a reason. I knew that if I were not where I was at that particular time, that in a few months I probably would have been dead, out on the street, away from my children, isolated from my family. I reflected on my concept of God. Even though I had chucked my Catholicism years before, I still had a trust that God existed, but not to help me. When my father lay in a coma, we prayed out loud as a family. I know it brought peace to my father because it was reflected on his face as he was dying. Accepting, watching death progress gave me a new insight into the meaning of life."

She remembered the day in his room discussing her problem with alcohol when she was so hung over and sick.

"He knew this was one thing his super overachiever daughter could not do on her own. I can remember his hurt look when I said I'd try AA. He knew I needed more to get through my thick intellectual head if I was going to survive. I realized, too, that my alcoholism was much like his cancer – incurable, hideous, self-destructive and humiliating. How strong he always was through life. How helpless he was in the last stages of cancer. Here I was with a terminal illness that could be arrested, procrastinating and acting like I had the answer. He always said I was so much like him, that what we do we do well, that our interests carry us far beyond the average person. The fear that alcohol would rob me of what I wanted to do in life began to erode my denial. I began to listen not only to others, but to the voice, the truth, inside me."

The fact that everyone in her family knew she was a drunk somehow made it easier to accept the fact that she had to change her way of life.

"I saw it as a relief, a release, a big green 'GO' for doing a lot of other things in life...I made the resolution to give myself over completely, to get home as soon as possible, but well enough to proceed with my future. There was still fear of what lay ahead, but each day without alcohol gave me more courage to change what I COULD change – ME."

The beauty of the lake was overwhelming this morning, like a scene from a Gothic novel. Not a ripple, the distant homes shrouded by tall green trees in summer now naked to the call of winter...the reflections of the boats dragged upon shore, of the red-roofed house across the way balancing the picture with a tree still clinging to its red-brown leaves, feathery reflections on the lake...wispy sky with streaks of blue and thin clouds layer upon layer...the bright red berries on the tree outside my room against the blue of my daughter's eyes in my precious photo of her...how I miss the children! I would love to take them for a walk in the woods and show them how the purple thistle bushes have turned brown but are still prickly, how the evergreens have not lost their brilliant greens.

Angie's journal October 28

Another event took place that Sunday that reinforced the shaky planking of Angie's new path. It was Family Day. Many of her "inmates" had visitors: husbands, siblings, children. Seeing their smiles with loved ones made her happy for them but a bit envious because her children were so far away.

"I talked with my husband and found that he had made arrangements to come to the family program, that he had done some soul-searching and wanted to look at his own drinking habits," she said. "I made an entry in my journal that he had explained to our eight year old son that 'mommy was at a place that will help her not become so upset all the time.' We talked about 'getting our shit together' as a family unit without dependence on alcohol. As I hung up I thought that his coming to the treatment center was a pretty scary thought. What if we no longer liked each other, let alone loved each other? Who were we, anyway, without alcohol?"

I am willing to accept whatever happens in the future and actually am looking forward to a new type of life, even though I have a lot of learning, reading, talking and soul-searching ahead of me. The dandelions have wilted and the milkweed is about to burst in my collection from outdoors...I wish I knew the names of all the different plants.

Angie's journal October 28

Angie recalls that getting sober was tiring, draining, wrenching those first few days.

"I didn't crave a drink, but my whole body was exhausted from adjusting to its new routine. Even after an afternoon nap I had difficulty in focusing on the program of lectures, exercise, meals. I never considered myself an addict, but after listening to the analysis of drugs and alcohol, I remembered how I had reacted to drugs during labor with my first child and how my family doctor had so compassionately given me Valium to 'calm my nerves' right before the beginning of the end of my drinking. I decided not to take the little pills because they made me so sleepy I couldn't drink and that's what I REALLY wanted. I also realized maybe there should be a place for 'potaholics' as my younger siblings all thought pot was the answer to their numerous problems. My middle brother, in a phone conversation, bared his soul about putting down pot when I went into treatment. He said maybe big Sis could do it for the rest of them so they wouldn't have to...well, maybe!"

On October 29 two new people joined Angie and the others on the unit. She was no longer the "new" person. She also had the thought about how ridiculous it was to actually be happy to be a little higher up in the pecking order in treatment! A few days without alcohol and she was still alive.

"I picked up the Prayer of St. Francis that day. It was my mother's favorite and was printed on my father's funeral card," she said "The prayer gave me a bit of solace from my childhood."

Lord, make me an instrument of Thy peace. Where there is hatred, let me sow love, where there is injury, pardon, where there is despair, hope, where there is doubt, faith, where there is darkness, light, where there is sadness, joy.

Oh Divine Master, grant that I may not so much seek to be consoled as to console, to be understood as to understand, to be loved as to love.

For it is in giving that we receive, it is in pardoning that we are pardoned and it is in dying that we are born to eternal life.

"I began to feel the old me dying," she recalled. "I felt like a new person looking at life, emotions and challenges. I felt like an infant. I begged God to please help me.

It was at that point that Angie was introduced to the first three steps of Alcoholics Anonymous and was asked to apply them to her own life.

"Because I never went to jail, never was arrested and had avoided being institutionalized, I had difficulty seeing how my life was unmanageable. I still had my business, the dog, the kids, the husband, the two cars, the house…yet my life *must* be a mess or I wouldn't be where I was."

Goblins and ghosties and Vern and Genny and Larry…we're finally rolling! I finally feel like there is some direction, like Group has finally come together. I'm getting punchy on all the good vibes from everyone in the family. Sometimes wish I didn't have all this support crap but how wonderful, really. Kids did okay in their ghost costumes I made before coming here and they promised to save the leftover peanut butter cups.
                                                Angie's journal October 31

At this time in treatment, Angie and the other women were introduced to the Big Book and the 12 Steps of Alcoholics Anonymous. There was resistance. Angie and some of the other women who were voluntarily in treatment still had the image of an old man in a trench coat under a bridge as the classic alcoholic. Now they all looked at each other as alcoholics, reflecting on why they were in treatment.

"I wasn't excited about examining the elements of Step One," she admitted. "I had never considered myself 'powerless,' yet I was asked to see how this step applied to my life."

Step One was divided into two parts.

We admitted we were powerless over alcohol...

It was such a simple word, powerless, but how did it apply to Angie?

"I was told to break the concept of powerless into seven areas of my life, including work, health, finances, reputation, relationships, education and self-respect," she said. "I scoffed at the idea of 'homework' but knew that if I wanted to complete treatment and get out of there I had better comply."

From the horrendous stories she heard from others on the unit it was easy to determine that she was what they called a 'high bottom' drunk.

"Never mind that I wanted to kill myself," she said, "and then there were all the 'yets.' I had not YET had a DUI. I had not YET ended in jail. I had not YET..."

Somehow she knew in her heart that getting sober would save her life, but she didn't know exactly how it would work. She didn't want the "yets" to happen. She knew they would ultimately lead her to death.

Work

Angie shuffled though her papers from treatment looking for her 'homework' on the first step. She stared at them for a moment, then said, "I am asked to examine how my use of alcohol affected my work. Having my own business I always thought I was in control. If I was hung over, I just moved an appointment to a later time, or came up with some lame excuse as to why I couldn't talk or meet or make a deadline for a promised project. It was more than procrastination. It was protecting my disease, consciously or unconsciously. I could manipulate hours or delegate some work I would normally do to my secretary."

She said she remembered having some difficulty trying to recall a specific incident to write about, but then chuckled.

"One night a client called about midnight. My husband answered the phone and was explaining to him that I couldn't come to the phone. I awoke out of a semi-sleep, or I may have passed out – who knows. I came into the office, took the phone from my husband and declared, 'I'm really not the troll under the bridge.' I handed the phone back to my husband who stood there dumfounded on what to say to cover up THAT one, and went back to bed."

She ended the segment on work with:

I know that if I continue to drink, my business will be seriously affected. I don't want to lose something I've worked so hard for.

Angie's Step One assignment

Health

Angie passed her physical at the treatment center and was told she was in good shape, that she had stopped drinking in time. But she reflected on whether or not she was taking care of herself prior to entering treatment.

"I had a pain beneath my right shoulder that felt like a knife in my back, a chronic pain that lasted for a year into sobriety," she said. "I knew it was tension, but if I drank enough I could numb the pain and pretend it wasn't there. After getting sober this solution was gone."

One thing Angie couldn't deny were her hangovers.

"I would open my eyes one at a time in the morning after drinking the night before, and if the sunlight didn't give me an instant headache, I would slowly raise my head and sit up," she said, going through the motion as she spoke. "I would ponder my condition before doing anything very quickly. Sometimes my head would pound, sometimes I would have to hang my head in the toilet. I could never predict the outcome of the night before, no matter if I had a whole bottle or a few sips of wine to go to sleep. It was always one or the other. I either tried to control the amount I drank or didn't give a damn how much I had."

Finances

"I know now that I didn't have a clue what they meant by looking at my financial situation," she said. "I arrogantly complained about the money spent on my treatment and added this to my homework:"

I do not feel I would have made more due to drinking or spent less.

Angie's Step One assignment

But she did admit that

I can see where financially I could be in jeopardy in the future, that drinking will eventually destroy what we've managed to build.

Angie's Step One assignment

Years later she said she would have rewritten the whole section on financial responsibility.

"If I had saved the cost of every bottle of alcohol I had bought over the years, I could have retired at an early age, or had one hell of a good time," she said. "The hours robbed that could have been billed, the contacts that were made and never followed up on, the jobs a healthy person could have pursued. The 'yets' can also work the other way around."

Reputation

Trying to see herself as others saw her was difficult for Angie.

"I arrogantly viewed myself as a party girl, as someone who got a lot of laughs from others when I drank. But I also noted how I was careful not to have a drink during a business lunch as I knew I couldn't just have one. There were times when my husband would escort me out of a meeting if I had joined in with a couple of cocktails to caution me to 'watch it.' Of course this always fueled resentment and defiance. Who was he (my business partner) to tell me how to behave in business?"

She said she never saw the consequences of her drinking until after she got sober and people commented on how "different" she was and how nice all the changes were.

"It made me angry, because I really liked the old me in a comfortable sort of way," she said. "It took a lot of time for me to realize the old me *wasn't* me, and that I now had the freedom to become the person I was *supposed* to be all along."

Relationships with Family and Others

Angie laughed looking at her notes.

"They could have just titled this one 'resentments,'" she said, noting that her writing was filled with blame on others: her husband, her children, her live-in help who left, her father for dying.

"I couldn't really write anything about 'others' as I had few friends by the time I entered treatment. Most had pleaded with me to do something about my drinking and I dismissed them as people who were jealous of me or who just didn't understand," she said. "Not having a close friend at the end of my drinking hit me hard: I had always maintained friendships with college friends and even a friend from high school, but at the point of entering treatment it was years since I had made any contact with them."

She remembers making a promise to herself to look up some of the old friends upon her return home, which she did, in fact, do. They are still her friends today, and with email, they are closer than ever.

Education

When Angie looked at what she had written on how

drinking had affected her education, she completely forgot about her college years and how drinking had put her on probation because of a low grade point average and prevented her from being on the sailing team.

"That should have been so obvious," she said. "It even affected how I helped my children with their school work. I was much more interested in drinking than taking the extra time with them, yet I was the first to say how important a good education was for my children."

Instead, she focused on her flight training, which she took a year before getting sober.

"On one occasion, I arrived for a lesson extremely hung over. I made some excuse to a rather tough instructor about 'having a fight with my husband' and canceled the training that day. I was so hung over I knew I had no business sitting left seat. Learning to fly at that point in my life really showed me that God was already doing for me what I could not do for myself. I learned to fly to conquer my fear of flying. When I got sober I became terrified once again and it took a year for me to get the courage to pilot again."

She also mentioned her six-month lag in reading *National Geographic*.

"It's funny how something so simple can reveal how out of character we have become at the end of our drinking," she said. "Looking back, I have so much more awareness today. My perceptions are different and I can be totally honest with myself."

Self-Respect

"Since I was so deeply into denial on how others saw me, I could only speculate on what they really thought," said Angie. "I know I was arrogant, haughty and self-important.

But I also know I was filled with self-loathing and doubt as to how 'good' I really was in all areas of my life. I lived in fear that you might find out how 'bad' I really was, how I was a total phony, projecting one person while being another."

Angie said her life had become one big coverup, a charade, a game of being what others wanted her to be. She said what others expected her to say, did what others expected her to do.

"I was in total survival mode, afraid that if I really looked at who I was I might not even exist," she said. "I might already be dead before I discovered how to live."

Then they examined the second half of Step One.

...that our lives had become unmanageable.

Angie, who thought she had always been in control of her life, soon realized that almost every aspect of her life was, after all, unmanageable. She shook her head, recalling her response at group when they asked her to talk about how her life was out of control.

"I coyly said, 'Excuse me, but I think I've managed quite well under all of these awful circumstances.'"

She said there was dead silence and a lot of blank stares.

"I had no clue on how unmanageable my situation had become. Although pressures of the business should have dictated I stop drinking, I continued. Although my anger level was frightening me with how I reacted to my children, I continued drinking. If my husband complained about my drinking, I drank on the sly, denying how much I consumed."

She mentioned her feelings of self-pity, resentment,

oversensitivity to criticism and that horrible pending fear and anxiety that ruled her life.

"When I finally looked at the big picture of my drinking, I could no longer intellectualize that my life was manageable," she said. "It was a mess. Pride transformed a sense of inferiority into a display of arrogance that kept me isolated in my mind and with others."

Now, in treatment, she was told that everything had to do with her, not with others. That it was Angie who created all these circumstances, that it was Angie's problem and that she needed to ask for help.

"Imagine," she smiled ironically. "Me ask for help? The controller who always knew what was best for everyone else without anyone asking for my expert advice? The one who drank every night to cope with the day, who lived in fear of being found out? Managing quite well? No way. When I finally realized what a mess my life REALLY was it was like a deck of cards falling. I began to see how it was all due to my drinking."

Her counselor asked her to write a paper titled "My Way."

"I soon concluded that My Way was No Way. The New Way would lead to Some Way."

Angie said there was humor in the collective despair of women getting sober. She recounted some of the stories, many from women she wouldn't think of associating with prior to treatment.

Karen told of watering down her husband's gin and not understanding why he was always so grumpy. She always made sure all the bottles in the garage were full. Never mind that they were full of water. It looked like she wasn't drinking. She often was invited with her successful husband to parties, where she would urinate wherever she happened to be sitting. He would get disgusted and periodically drive her to the local detox where she'd stay in her nightgown for five days.

Gail, with a husband and three sons, stashed her liquor bottles in Kotex boxes. Another talked about drinking Cepacol and aftershave. Barb stashed her booze behind the canned goods in the pantry. One day she discovered her kids had put a skull and crossbones on the bottles. Another talked about purchasing something on her credit card, returning it without the sales slip, and getting cash to spend on booze. The purchase showed up on the statement to account for the missing money. Connie, an ex-nun chemistry teacher, bragged about making LSD in the lab (lions, snakes and dragons).

And then there was Carol, who walked around in a daze. She had lived with her mother all her life and started drinking at 50 after her mother's death. Her sister, a nun, didn't know what to do with her so dumped her at the treatment center.

Sharon, on drugs since the age of three and now 28, had to be carted off in a seizure to the hospital to help her through withdrawals. Her doctor father had used her to experiment with drugs while her mother doled out tranquilizers and sleeping pills...the list of what she had been given was endless.

Mary, who signed over her last nickel to come to treatment at the age of 53, was placed in extended care after several relapses and climbing out of the slums, one of triplets in a family of eight kids.

And Ellen, sweet little woman at 63 whose husband lived on Antabuse in a trailer.

"We were all ages, from all economic backgrounds,

some highly educated and others unable to read," said Angie. "We were helpless, lonely sisters in grief, despair and hopelessness. Together we pooled our strengths and weaknesses, our fears and dreams. We all longed for a better life. We all craved happiness and contentment. We all knew there had to be a better way to live. We prayed that the miracle would happen."

For the first time, Angie said she felt kinship with other women, that she belonged, that maybe something magical would happen to make her life better, happier.

This place is really volatile. Up and down, in and out. You never know who is the next one to implode or explode. It is colder every day, so I go out less. A card from my mother lifted me: "I thought of you the other day and by golly, the sun came up...and the next day I thought of you and the flowers sprouted on the land...and the day after that I thought of you and the beasts walked in the field...and when I thought of you the next day the rains came down...and the next day the rains poured forth from the heavens...and when I thought of you the day after that, the birds sang. Today I rested. What's new with you?" She writes of canning and juicing and woodworking and auto mechanics...what energy that woman has...the realization of dad's death still hangs, although she has a grasp on it...I know she must ache inside, but she'll always show strength to the world and us kids.
Angie's journal November 4

Then Angie's group was ready to examine Step Two.

Came to believe that a power greater than ourselves could retore us to sanity.

Raised Catholic, Angie said her "power greater than ourselves" was God.

"But God ceased to exist for me as my alcoholism progressed in the early stages," she said. "I can remember the first time I refused to go to Sunday Mass. I was 21, hung over, and arrived late in the choir loft of the little school chapel. Service was well under way. The nun at the organ stood and glared at me, her fingers frozen on the keys, telling me to 'go down in front.' I mentally said 'f... you' and left. I wandered along the river from one end of the campus to the other. Surely God understood. Surely He didn't want to see me humiliated. Surely it really didn't matter in the greater scheme of things whether I went to Sunday church or not."

After that it was easy for her to shrug off Mass, and as time went on, Angie not only stopped going to church, she also stopped praying. After all, she reasoned, if God really loved her, why would she feel so awful all the time, emotionally and physically? Surely she had been forgotten.

"It was at this point in treatment that I was told I could move to the private room I had made such a fuss about in the beginning.," she said. "By that time I was comfortable with my roommate and really didn't relish the thought of being isolated."

She had no choice.

"They just repeated that my room was ready," she said, shrugging her shoulders. "I grudgingly carried my belongings to a small cubbyhole of a room and settled in, but the anger and resentment were evident. I was not a contented camper."

Then discussion in group explored the concept of sanity. What exactly did it mean?

"I knew I was crazy and actually preferred being crazy

to being alcoholic, but if I was to get through this step it meant doing some introspective work," said Angie. "I reflected on the God of my childhood, on my 16 years of Catholic education. I really knew nothing about God. But something or some force had brought me to my knees, had led me to the door of recovery."

Her first conscious spiritual awakening came late one afternoon. She was sitting in her little room looking out to the lake, the trees and the grounds. There was a light snow falling, the trees stark against a grey sky. Little patches of leftover green poked through snow covered beds along the buildings and walkways. It was bleak but beautiful.

"It just hit me," said Angie. "It was so simple! Sanity was order. Insanity was disorder. Everything in God's universe had order. The sun came up every morning. The stars lit up the heavens. It rained or snowed on a regular basis. Ants built their hill and went about their busy life every day. Bears hibernated every winter. Flowers bloomed every spring. Here I was, a mere human being, OUT OF ORDER with God's universe. HE didn't make me an alcoholic. I became one of my own free will. Never mind all the genetic causes and people who could be blamed for the process. This step promised me I could regain sanity, that there could be order in my life, that I could walk in rhythm with the universe, a simple, unimportant cog in God's wheel of life. It was such a simple, yet divine concept."

Later in her sobriety, Angie often referred to that moment in Step Two as her first significant spiritual awakening. It allowed her to be open for the next step.

Sanity is peace of mind, with a warm feeling in the heart that I have not hurt anyone on a day-to-day basis. Sanity is rational thinking, consideration of others, trust in God and confidence in myself. Sanity means living a sober, fulfilling life. I've seen such tremendous change in so many around me. I believe I can restore my life to one filled with happiness, love and work well done. I believe because I WANT to believe.

Self Assessment, Step Two

"After writing this, I played my guitar for awhile, experiencing a new contentment," she said. "It was the first time I felt I was going to be all right. I was going to survive. I was going to somehow start over, or go back to where I had screwed up. I knew I was being given a second chance. I knew that, despite my journey of anguish, God still loved me. He had brought me to that little room, to see His orderly universe, to reflect on the path ahead."

And then, Step Three:

Made a decision to turn our will and our lives over to the care of God as we understood Him.

Because of her Catholic upbringing, Angie was convinced that God really didn't care about her anymore.

"I had chucked all that He had stood for, or so I thought, but part of me longed to have the God of my childhood back," she said.

She often hears other recovering Catholics talk about their "punishing" God.

"Because my mother had such a hard-rock faith (she's now a Baptist) I was always taught that God was there to help me," she said. "My alcoholism robbed me of this knowledge because in order to get help I knew I had to ask for it. How could God help me when I had gotten myself into such a mess? Many times I blamed God for abandoning me, for making my life miserable. So, when it came to doing the Third Step I didn't know if God was going to be there for me."

She explained that in the difficult growing up years, pre-teen through about 16, she often found herself sitting on the rectory steps of her church waiting for the parish priest to have time to rescue the family.

"There was a lot of turmoil at home that I didn't understand at the time, and only through treatment can I reflect on the dysfunction," she said. "When I hear about the physical, mental and emotional abuse many recovering women had to deal with in their childhood, I almost feel guilty mentioning dysfunction in my family. It was a supportive, encouraging, loving home. The ONLY time there was ever a problem was when too much alcohol was consumed. It was at these times that Father Tom would step in and referee, a priest who helped alcoholics in the parish, who never drank anything in our home at that time except coffee."

Angie shook her head, then told how Father Tom, unfortunately, had to experience his "yets." She said he volunteered for Viet Nam and years later visited their home and drank Scotch. Eventually he left the priesthood, married a divorcee and ultimately died of alcoholism.

"He was God's representative for our family in those early years, and the memories of his help and genuine concern for us reflect a loving, not punishing God," said Angie. "It grieves me to think of him dying of this disease when he seemed to have such a grasp on the program at one time. It tells me that it IS progressive, and that every sober day is a gift."

To me, God is Chairman of the Board. Although decisions are made at a lower level of competency by me, it is through

His direction these decisions are made, acted upon through relationships with others for the benefit of me and those concerning me. I may not know the total outcome of His plan, nor do I question His motives. I only do my best to cooperate and trust.

Self Assessment, Step Three

In treatment, Angie talked about "will" being a day-to-day occurrence, with "life" being an overall plan, and that it is the combination of all the "wills" that makes up "life."

"I reasoned that by turning over my will, my life's plan according to my Higher Power would automatically follow," she said.

As someone who was always in control, she found herself becoming more compliant.

"I actually felt relief as I went through self-examination and acceptance of this step," she said. "I began feeling less responsible for everyone around me, I became more relaxed, easygoing and open to suggestions from others, something I bitterly fought at the beginning of treatment. I initially questioned how these strangers could possibly identify with my feelings. How could they understand my lifestyle in Florida, my particular problems with family, business and relationships? Didn't they know how different I am?"

She said she found alcohol to be the leveler, that there is nothing unique about one alcoholic.

"The only difference is whether we receive the grace to get sober or if we are left to die of our disease," she said. "Those seeking recovery are all climbing out of the same black hole looking for relief, for a new life. We have all felt we were crazy, misunderstood, vulnerable. We have all felt anger, anguish, despair. We have all been brought to our knees to ask for help."

I am tired of trying to control and feel relief that I have changed direction. The day I knew I could no longer control my drinking and asked for help was the turning point. It allowed me to return to God. In turning over my will, my mind is open, ready for options.
Self Assessment, Step Three

Angie's spiritual advisor in treatment entered the ministry after being an advertising executive, so she intuitively knew he had her number when it came to being honest and telling her story. He would show up whenever she had group or discussion, and often caught her in some public relations ploy that had nothing to do with the truth of her recovery.

"One day in the hallway I was moaning and groaning about something as he passed by and he said, 'Step Three.' I replied 'Piss on Step Three.' He said, 'Step One.' And so it went," she smiled. "A couple of steps forward, a step back. Intellectually I understood what was being taught and what I had to do, but my instincts were to challenge every concept, to question, to have a better idea, to criticize and compare."

Since the psychological and mental tests they administered to Angie showed she still had all her brain power, she thought why not use it? But she soon realized that Step Three had nothing to do with being "right" or smart.

"It had everything to do with surrendering my old ways, to being open to a God who could lead me through life's circumstances," she said. "It meant getting out of my own way, quieting my mind. It meant asking God every day to help me recognize His will, then to accept it and follow through. It was so simple, sometimes impossible, but always successful. I no longer had to make all those decisions. I just had to follow through and not worry about the consequences. If it was the right thing to do, then right actions would follow. The right people would be put in my path. They would speak the wisdom of the God of my understanding. I just had to listen."

God, grant me the Serenity to Accept the things I cannot change, Courage to change the things I can, and Wisdom to know the difference.

As the Serenity Prayer became part of her daily routine, Angie realized there was little she could change except herself.

"One of the biggest lessons was that no one can 'do' anything to me unless I allow it," she said. "If I'm angry at someone I have to look at myself. What has this triggered? Where is the REAL source of this anger? If I feel less-than or superior-to any person or situation, it is not THEM, it's ME I have to look at. It often means simple acceptance, no more, no less. God's plan will proceed with or without me. And He works in other people's lives as well as mine."

Over the years, she said Step Three was a lifesaver for "getting off the hook." She found it easier as the years went on to incorporate Step Three and God's will as a way of life.

"I'm not saying I listen to that quiet voice all the time," she said. "But it changed my perception of life. I'm just one more ant in the hill doing what God wants me to do to the best of my human ability. When I think something is good for me, I step back and see if I have any thoughts or reaction to the contrary. It's amazing how Step Three can work when, as they say in meetings, you work it."

Next, the group began the journey exploring Step Four, often the stumbling block for alcoholics still in doubt or denial.

Made a searching and fearless moral inventory of ourselves.

Angie was familiar with the Catholic sacrament of Penance, and when she came to Steps Four and Five, she had visions of the confessional, of a priest giving her absolution along with a few "Hail Marys."

"As I sat in my room staring at my typewriter to start Step Four I didn't know where to begin," she said. "It was overwhelming. I had several guide pamphlets, the Big Book and thoughts from group on how others began, but nothing seemed to help me get started."

Being given a deadline helped, and today Angie recommends to sponsees that they also set a time limit. She feels that procrastination can be a rationalized convenience for an alcoholic not wanting to face the truth.

"The more I fought doing this step, though, the more difficult it became," she said. "I knew in order to stay sober I had to find out what was behind my disease. I had to explore my feelings, my resentments, my fears. I had to see that it wasn't 'them' but 'me' that caused any problem. Again, people don't 'do' things to me – I allow myself to react to people and situations."

Because Angie mostly drank at home, she said her fourth step primarily focused on family and close personal and business relationships.

"I hadn't stolen money from anyone, but I had certainly stolen time, which in business IS money," she said.

It was important to constantly remind herself that Step Four is an inventory.

"It isn't just all the bad things in my life, but also the good things," she said. "I was encouraged to write the positive as well as the negative, even if I could just admit that I'm a good cook or seamstress, or that I could give someone a nice smile."

She began digging for the little things that she once liked about herself, a bit difficult at first because she admitted she had developed such self loathing in the course of her disease.

"Balancing resentments with good memories, unacceptable behavior with acts of kindness and fears with positive action and faith helped me develop an inventory with liabilities offset by assets," she said. "I also gave God credit for giving me an incredible amount of talent."

Angie's only regret was that she burned Step Four after doing Step Five.

"It was the fashionable thing to do in treatment at the time," she explained, "sort of a ritual. I actually had a difficult time lighting a match to my pile of papers and getting them to burn because there was so much snow on the ground. I wished later that I had all those papers for the eighth step because I had to recall a lot of that information. I now encourage anyone who takes the time to do all the work in Step Four to save it for later, but hide it in a secret place. It's not something you want your kids or spouse to find."

Angie said she did another Step Four at seven years sober, but that one focused on her relationship with all the men in her life – her father, her brothers and other family members, boyfriends, her husband – men in general.

"I had no idea how I was programmed to be a people-pleaser while harboring resentments, particularly as a woman who started her own business before it was fashionable," she said. "There were many obstacles created by men in those early days that I had to overcome. Until I did this step, writing in detail how I felt about the men in various stages of my life, I was unable to see the resentments, along with the justification to drink, that had grown over a long period of time. I was eventually able to view men as people who, even though most didn't want to admit it, also had feelings."

She developed self respect to avoid acting out of "duty" or selfishness sexually and to comfortably conduct herself without compromising principles in friendship and business.

"In the past I always felt I had to justify what I was doing or what I was charging professionally. I learned that it's okay to just do what I have to do and charge what I feel is right," she said.

She also adopted the acronym "**JADE**" that tells her she doesn't have to *justify*, *apologize*, *defend* or *explain* anything.

"I can just say 'yes' or 'no' in any situation," she said. "I always thought I had to give a reason why I felt the way I did, which would open my feelings to discussion. One word answers are okay today."

Then it was time for Step Five, often dreaded by newcomers to sobriety. What they learn, however, is that this step leads to freedom – of self, of the past. It opens the door to happiness and being comfortable. It's the beginning of finding out who we really are and it allows us to forgive.

Admitted to God, to ourselves, and to another human being the exact nature of our wrongs.

Angie felt fortunate to share Step Five with a spiritual advisor who coached her through Step Four during treatment, but, she emphasized, it did not make it any easier. If anything, she couldn't cover up or avoid issues.

"By the time I got to this step I had stopped blaming God for getting me into my alcoholic predicament and really believed and trusted that He was working in my life," she said. "So, taking my inventory to God was not difficult. Looking at myself honestly and objectively was a bigger challenge, and sharing all this with another person was a bit overwhelming. I remember crying and being consoled that I had done the best I could under the circumstances, and I learned that I was not a bad person becoming good but a sick person becoming well through the process."

When it was all over she truly felt she had a clean slate, that she could start living life the way God wanted her to all along.

"I was able to forgive myself and others." She chuckled and shook her head, recalling the burning of her fourth step. "When the flame finally took I actually smiled as my list of resentments went up in smoke. I felt peace and relief. I had given myself permission to begin again."

Angie said she is grateful for the guidance she received through Steps Four and Five and highly recommends that these steps be done with a spiritual advisor or sponsor.

"I also feel strongly that the steps be done in order," she said. While I did the first five during treatment, I was encouraged to begin Step Six with a sponsor upon 're-entry.' At first I was overwhelmed with day-to-day living situations, but as soon as possible, I resumed the steps because with each one, my sobriety became stronger, I was happier and life became easier as alcohol no longer ruled my life."

Because she was so ignorant of alcoholism and the treatment process, Angie said she feels it's important to share her journey with other women to alleviate their fears and to give them courage to recover.

"Other women know in their heart, like I did, that they

are alcoholic and need help, whether it means going through treatment or having the courage to walk through the doors of AA. There are women all over the world who got sober with the help of other women who have gone before them. It's not important HOW we get sober, only that we DO!"

As treatment progressed, Angie was asked to explore her feelings.

"I had ignored them for so long, drowning them in alcohol, that I felt dead inside," she said. "Many times I felt hurt with no one to turn to. I felt the burden of decision making. It seemed like it was easier on everyone in the family if I decided what should be done, but I later felt cheated out of support I feel I should have had."

Angie quietly talked about how her love for music, always an escape, was squashed in her home. Her husband claimed to be "tone deaf" and never related to her music, classical or otherwise. He complained it was "too loud," so her reaction was to turn it off altogether and stuff another layer of resentment.

She shook her head. "I would just have a drink and forget about it, a pattern that was repeated in all areas of my life. If someone didn't understand me, I found it almost impossible to explain myself. I didn't know what was causing my reaction, only that it made me angry and frustrated. It was easier to put another brick in my wall to hide me from having to deal with it."

Ironically, she was able to function on levels of business, making decisions, paying bills, scheduling appointments (but not always keeping them if she had a hangover), getting the children to school on time, being an involved parent and running the house.

"I couldn't understand how other people found it difficult to function," she said. "If I could do it drinking the way I did, surely they could do it under normal circumstances."

One of the character traits she has always found difficult to deal with is procrastination.

"This is a huge control issue for me," she said. "When I get an idea in my head, I usually follow through. When there is a problem in business, I try to solve it immediately. There were many times prior to recovery that I drank because my partner or someone else didn't follow through collecting money, scheduling appointments or making phone calls. It drove me crazy, but my solution was always the same: drown my feelings in alcohol and hope that things would change. Of course they didn't. I learned in recovery that if nothing changes, nothing changes. My solution not only made me feel alone, it also propelled me into incredible loneliness. Alcohol alienated me from everyone who could possibly touch this loneliness."

She turned the page in her journal, looking at what she had written:

Have verbalized my frustrations, anger and resentment (stir in a little self-pity) and will now shelve this concoction and try to move on. I'm feeling really down, but I have a beautiful bouquet of dried leaves, milkweed and miscellaneous weeds to brighten the room. I still feel like playing the guitar and singing, and I'm thankful for a lot of things, like the blue jay that visited outside today.
Angie's journal, November 15

Because there were alcoholics in her life, Angie was urged to attend the family program at the treatment center, sort of a crash course in Al-Anon, which extended her personal treatment for a few more days.

"By the second day I felt myself defending my disease. It was impossible to convey to the non-chemically dependent person the disease of alcoholism," she said, shaking her head. "I heard terms like 'weakness' and 'will power' and 'morality.' As family members shared, I was overcome with a sense of sadness and the realization of how insidious this disease is to everyone connected to the alcoholic."

Her therapist began preparing her for "re-entry," as if she were going to break through a huge barrier and descend upon the living as one of "them" once again.

"It was difficult making calls to assure help would be there and for me to attend meetings as soon as possible. In discussing my fears with my counselor, I remember a gnawing feeling when talking about my family. I missed my children terribly and couldn't wait to hold them in my arms, to comfort them, to enjoy them," she said, "but I did not have that same feeling concerning my husband. I had an overwhelming fear that I may have to end my marriage in order to stay sober."

When her counselor told Angie her chances of staying sober were slim – that she was too smart, too analytical, and her bottom too "high" – the defiance that brought her to treatment became an asset.

"I told her, 'I'll show you!' It was a spontaneous reaction," she said, "but inside I had doubts. How could I possibly survive going home and not drinking? My drinking buddy husband was now sober a few weeks. Did I even know who he was? Did I ever know?"

As Angie's recovery journal ends her life begins again. Seeing her little family as she stepped off the plane was "wonderful but strange."

"In that short time we were all different people," she

said. "Instead of feeling secure and happy, I was terrified. I wondered how I was going to live. I felt thrust out of the womb, but this time with all the knowledge of the world and my choices. One side of me wanted to run back to my room at treatment, to be cared for, nourished and protected. I felt vulnerable, as if they had taken me totally apart, then glued me back together. I was home but the glue hadn't set. Would it ever?"

The First Year

The most difficult time in Angie's sobriety occurred in the first and seventh years. The first year enlightened her about who she was, but it took a year for her to laugh again, to be comfortable in her own skin, to take herself less seriously, and to give others the space they needed for themselves.

"The first four months found me at morning meetings at the local halfway house for women alcoholics," she said, shaking her head as she recalled the small smoke-filled room with rescued furnishings. "It was the only place I felt safe to sob through a meeting. If I needed feedback, I could get it, but mostly I just cried, identifying with the feelings of so many women struggling to live again. It was a safe haven, away from my family. I was just a face, just another desperate, confused woman trying to put her life back together. It amazed me how comfortable I became in those meetings, like they were an extension of treatment. It was the most important hour of my day."

In the evening she usually attended meetings at a local recovery clubhouse, and the "Why it Works" group became her home group. It explored both the 12 Steps of AA for personal recovery, and the 12 Traditions, the foundation for groups.

As Angie got "better" she also noticed that the family was healing. There was more caring, more tenderness, more understanding, less arguing, more routine.

"My children, ages 4 and 8, learned the Serenity Prayer and about making amends if they did or said something to hurt someone," she said. "We were integrating the principles of AA into our home life. While I went to my meetings, my husband went to his, but we rarely went together. I don't know if this set the theme for the difficult seventh year or not, but I treasured my meetings and would not have felt comfortable sharing in his presence. I'm sure he felt the same."

Getting an AA sponsor (something she had promised her counselor she would do right away) was difficult at first, but Angie knew if she was to stay sober she had to find a woman she could call day or night, who could get to know her better than she knew herself.

"The first two women I asked declined, which was a blow to my ego," she said. "It took so much courage to ask anyone that it injured my fragile, new-found self-esteem when they gave me legitimate reasons why they couldn't sponsor me. But by the end of the first six months, I had a wonderful sponsor who helped me through the remaining steps, who had me speak at my first meeting at a year's sobriety, and who then dumped me (and everyone else) as she went off to become a minister when I was almost two years sober."

By that time, Angie knew enough recovering women that getting another sponsor was not a big deal, although she coasted for almost another year before asking Rita to be her sponsor.

"My home life was more difficult and I was getting more and more irritated and disillusioned with my marriage," she said. "It was made more difficult by the fact that we were also in business together. I still had my own business, but WE had a business and everything seemed so entwined that I found it difficult to separate business issues and problems from home issues and problems. I began to feel trapped 24 hours a day with someone I really didn't know any more, who in his own recovery had also changed. We drifted apart across the dining table, in the same office, wherever we went, pretending that all was well."

About the third year of sobriety and at her sponsor's urging, Angie suggested marriage counseling to her husband.

"Since he believed the only problem we had was sexual, me being the one at fault, I agreed to go to a sex therapist." She paused, then shook her head. "In hindsight I realize this narrowed any chance for solving the real problems with the marriage; that going along with his diagnosis was not in my best interest. After six sessions, with me dutifully following through with all the suggestions and actually having some fun with it, he abruptly stopped the appointments. When I asked him why all he said was, 'She isn't telling you what I wanted her to tell you.'"

Her sponsor said it was normal for men to view therapy as something for "the other person," that it was really a control issue.

"Had he agreed to marriage counseling instead, progress could have been made, but I never again could convince him that therapy might help the situation. So guess what?" she grinned. "I went on my own, paying for it out of my own pocket, on my own time schedule."

She chose a woman counselor who understood alcoholism. Angie began having identity and dignity and, most of all, faith that she could handle whatever lay ahead.

"My prayers were that God would work through my counselor to guide me to do whatever was necessary for my sobriety and well-being."

Living One Day At A Time Through The 12 Steps of Alcoholics Anonymous

Years in sobriety are not magic markers to color in the time of our lives, but tools to unveil the soul, one day at a time...sometimes seriously, always in earnest, but with enough whimsy to laugh at ourselves as we hold hands, skipping along the yellow brick road of recovery.

Angie's writings 1987

While the Big Book of Alcoholics Anonymous gives the best possible road map on recognizing alcoholism, getting and staying sober, it tends to be male oriented. In the early days, it was two men who started AA and the first to get sober were men. While there were a few women who got sober in the early days, it was not the norm. Over the years chapters have been added to the Big Book that women can identify with, but women getting sober today is different than men getting sober 60 years ago when the Book was originally written.

In the early days, the woman alcoholic was confined to her home, stealing booze from the household stock. She rarely went out to the bars and purchasing liquor was not the norm. That was the man's job. When the wife and mother of his children became alcoholic, the tendency was to keep her at home, out of sight and silent. The elephant (often used to symbolize alcoholism) was in the home, but everyone kept it well fed so it didn't have to venture very far and certainly not make any noise. Give the old lady a drink and shut her up.

Men have wanted control over women from time immemorial. It's the nature of the beast. If he could control her liquor, he could control her.

Angie believes the turning point for women came about 1966, the year she graduated college.

"It was the first time we told the boys at the university across the road that we didn't want to get married, sit home and have their children. We'd like to go to work, have a career and, of course, the right to drink."

Years later, following her divorce, she found that men much older than she were fine with everything she wanted to do because they had seen their daughters grow up in "the movement."

"Men ten years younger than I didn't have a clue on how it once was," she said. "They expected women to earn their own money and, of course, to drink. It is the men in my own age group that to this day struggle with the girls who told them to take a leap years ago. They never recovered from this mindset because they were never prepared or conditioned as young boy children for women to think on their own, have a career, make their own money or to drink on their own."

She feels that women's role, women's openness, women's drinking habits, and the availability of booze and pills have changed over the years, and in many ways, women in recovery are in direct proportion to their age group.

"We don't see as many women in the rooms of AA who could and should be in recovery," she said. "There are only a few older women in the program, and I don't think this is just the result of old age. Many women died of the disease before getting the chance to get sober, were sent to mental institutions, or retreated to the confines of their minds, their own little world, to mask their feelings and their disease."

She said there are more middle-aged women in the program because they grew up during the transition of women from homemakers to professionals/workers.

"It logically follows that the majority of women in AA today are young, meaning thirty-something or even younger," she said. "They were fortunate to grow up in an age when alcoholism was recognized as a disease of human beings, not just men, and when it was acceptable, sometimes even fashionable, to get treatment, to live life regardless of what the men in their lives thought."

She said women today can celebrate the emancipation of the woman alcoholic. She is finally free – to be, to get emotional help, to love and be loved. She is free to get sober. Hurray!

Still Sober

In reflecting back over the years, Angie doesn't know how so many one-day-at-a-times mushroomed into almost 30 years of continuous sobriety.

"The only answer I have is that God must love me very much," she smiled, pointing out that the homework for the lessons learned in those years has not been easy.

"Sometimes I dug in my heels and refused to move on, holding on to my own ideas. But there was always someone to encourage me, to offer a hand, to guide me through the step pertaining to the problem, to help me walk through the dark tunnel because THEY could see the light at the end."

What she has learned is how to live without drinking.

"It sounds so simple. Just don't drink...just say 'No,' she said, shaking her head. "But what happens when a relationship dies, a family crumbles, divorce looms? What happens when you lose a loved one, a partner, a child, a parent? Those were all reasons to drink in the past. Now what do you do?"

She continued with the list of day-to-today questions confronting the sober alcoholic: What happens when financial disaster strikes and the worry over paying bills (forget the long-range picture of saving for the future!) leaves you with anxiety and a grip on your insides that won't let up? What happens when your boss, in the midst of all this turmoil, gives you a pink slip and there's no money coming in at all? What happens when you almost reach retirement age and are set back by ill health related to years of drinking and abuse, with no insurance, waiting for age 65 to arrive so you can finally get the necessary tests done? How do you react when you are sober a number of years and the news media comes up with the "answer to alcoholism" that you KNOW would be fatal if followed? What do you do when you can no longer drink or pop a "happy pill"?

"On the other side," she asked, "how do you handle success? THAT's as good a reason to drink as failure. Celebrate with some bubbly! How do you handle more money than you've ever had without blowing it on expensive wine while you entertain important clients? Or, how do you entertain them while they drink and you do not? How do you toast your son or daughter at their wedding...or how do YOU go through your own ceremony without the usual toasts?"

She said those who take sobriety seriously, who work a daily spiritual program based on the 12 Steps of Alcoholics Anonymous, and who help other alcoholics must learn how to handle these situations.

"But it doesn't happen overnight, and today's sobriety is not a guarantee for tomorrow," she pointed out. "It is a day at a time, sometimes a minute at a time, pursuit of spiritual, mental, emotional and physical health."

She also emphasized that there is no "graduating," no "cure," no "answer to all."

"But sobriety is happiness," she said. "It returns us to sanity. It gives us our life back. It allows us to make choices. Sobriety is freedom...from the past, from our despair. Sobriety is a chance to start over, to become the person we were always supposed to be."

But how do we get there? How do we start on this journey and with each step get stronger, healthier, happier?

"I was told early on in sobriety that I had to change everything: how I thought, how I acted, how I behaved, how I treated others, how I treated myself," she said. "It meant setting boundaries, learning what was good for ME, not all the other people in my life that I was always concerned with in the past. It meant finding out the difference between being selfish and selfless and developing self-worth. It meant reprogramming, reaching back to the depths of my beginning to find out what God's plan was for me before booze put up the barrier, before alcohol crushed my emotional development and robbed me of my spirit."

When she entered treatment she didn't know that alcoholism is one of the top killers, yet a treatable disease. It wasn't until she got the "head" knowledge, documented with statistics and stories of recovery, that she was able to finally look at herself as she was – a woman with a fatal disease who really didn't want to die.

"But I also didn't know how to live," she said. "I had to find out from other women who had walked the journey, who helped each other become sober, happy, mentally and spiritually well women. I laughed with them at their 'God stories' and shared in their sorrows and struggles. But most of all, I accepted their gift of hope. I realized that I if I could learn how to live happily by listening to the women in AA, any woman could."

With Angie's guidance, we began exploring life situations, events that happen along life's path whether women are sober or still wondering what happened to them. We applied the 12 Steps to each of these situations with stories of how sober women dealt with them in real life.

Because alcohol is so disruptive to a stable family life, we began with one of the most devastating situations, one that often occurs just prior to getting sober or after recovery begins as a result of major changes taking place in both the individual getting sober and in the partner dealing with a "new" person.

Divorce

When Angie was in treatment, a sense of panic engulfed her during a session with her therapist that was so troubling she could only let the thought surface for a second before dismissing it as "impossible." But it began to recur and to visit her in the dead of sleep.

"It was the realization that I had married my drinking buddy," she said, "and that one of the reasons was to escape. I knew that if I were sober, I would be a different person. Although I didn't want to face reality, I knew, in the pit of my stomach and a special corner of my mind, that the marriage had a good chance of falling apart, but I made a commitment to myself to keep the family together as long as possible."

She spoke with many of her fellow "inmates" on their individual situations. Many marriages had broken up as a result of alcoholism, leaving a string of divorces and disappointments and confused children. In almost every case, the person ended up marrying another alcoholic or an abuser or someone similar to the previous relationship. It became a cycle that seemingly couldn't be broken, repeated again and again with the end result always the same.

One of the early slogans she learned and took to heart was "Nothing changes, nothing changes."

"The solution always involves changing myself – my attitude, my outlook, my own behavior," she said. "If I change, then the situation changes, regardless if the OTHER person makes any changes."

Angie's personal situation was compounded by both partners getting sober at the same time.

"While this could have been a win-win scenario, which happens with many sober couples, it was complicated by both of us growing in different ways, different directions, on a different spiritual timetable," she said. "Just stopping drinking was not the answer. We both went to many meetings, alternating nights so one parent could be home with the children, and we really tried to make the marriage work. Being in business together also posed complications. While we had a united front in running the business, our personal lives were deteriorating. There was tension, disagreement, finger pointing, misunderstanding, the pressure of deadlines and money matters wearing us down. The children were right in the middle, not knowing the 'mood' that would dictate the day."

She said that while they were both staying sober, she felt she was living with a "dry drunk," a difficult situation because booze can no longer be blamed for alcoholic behavior.

"We just progressed on a different timetable," she said. "The marriage hindered the full growth potential of us individually, as it was really over even though we both hung on."

Angie and her ex-husband now have a healthy relationship years after the divorce (she's even spoken for him when he was chairing an AA meeting!) and in accordance with Step Nine, her intention today is not to hurt or blame.

"In AA we learn that we are not unique, that our problems are shared with countless others in recovery, and that the solution for all situations is in working the Steps," she said.

Angie at first resented a fellow alcoholic who told her when she started pointing the finger of blame at her ex- that she could only hold him 50 percent responsible for the divorce.

"This was a hard pill to swallow and it took a long time for me to realize that we were on a seesaw, never in sync with each other, always at opposite ends," she said. "I also learned the most important lesson of all: I am responsible only for myself, no one else. I have no control over my partner's thoughts, behavior, personality, actions or reactions. I can do only what I am supposed to do for me, not for someone else. And I cannot predict or assume how anyone else will feel or act. In truth, it's none of my business."

She reflected on her feelings in the process leading to divorce, which occurred seven years into her sobriety, sharing what she did for herself to get through the turmoil, the emotional pain.

"One of the best tools was writing down my feelings, writing letters to the other person even though they were never meant to be sent, composing poetry that soothed my emotions," she said. "By qualifying MY thoughts and actions on paper, the situation became more real, more tangible, something that could be set aside as a separate entity to view objectively. Once in writing, I could then take the issues to my sponsor or to a trusted friend to help me sort matters out, to make the changes necessary for me to stay sober."

She admitted there were many times when she thought to pick up a drink – "I'll show HIM!"

"Then I would look at my children, realize that drinking was not an option and proceed with my own spiritual conditioning," she said. "I still go over my writings during difficult times in my life. These were written about a year prior to the divorce, expressing my feelings and frustration."

The same suicide thoughts as before sobriety have started to resurface...I can't cope with the unloving, fake, cruel atmosphere I feel trapped in. I'm torn between loving my children and hating my husband, but the thought of leaving them with him is enough to keep me going. I'm writing to go beyond my thoughts, to get me on the right track, knowing there is a God who loves me and for some goddamn reason has created this scene for me to weather. I know I am to grow by it but it is almost too much to handle at this point.

I was looking for some quiet time at the island, but unless I sit at the ocean beach all day I'm afraid I won't get it. I am selfish, angry and feeling totally unloved. If I could get out of this relationship this minute I would but I know that's not supposed to happen. I pray for the strength to get me through this and to use this hurt to good purpose. It's like a one-way street for me right now, but instead of backing up, I should be going forward, looking toward new horizons, a new sunrise and sunset.

This will pass, as it has before, and I know there will be more joy than ever before. I need to trust, to turn my life over so that I don't take it so personally, but my need for someone to hold me, to understand me, and just plain give a shit is so strong that I feel as fragile as an eggshell. I know I can't control someone else, that I can only change myself, but this change process is turning me around almost completely in my mind. I feel cramped, taken for granted, hurt and oh, so very, very alone and lonely. The only option I possess is prayer and my program, because I will break and shatter into a million pieces if I let my mind have its way.
Angie's writings 1985

At this point in Angie's sobriety, she was already in a step study group with several other women, including her sponsor.

"Because I felt so betrayed, resentful, angry and frustrated over the men who had been in my life, from my father to husband to brothers to friends, it was suggested I do a Fifth Step following a Fourth Step I did strictly on my relationships with the men," she said. "Because I am such a strong, powerful woman in terms of getting things done, organizing and controlling, I had a lot of looking inside to do."

She knew her feelings stemmed from men not doing what she expected, not giving her what she needed or wanted at the time or even doing a simple task she asked.

"It was pointed out that someone can't give what they don't have, whether it be emotional support, love or even security," she said. "I came to realize that because I outwardly portrayed a very together, headstrong, competent woman, the vulnerable, soft side of me was never seen. I guarded it and protected it. How could anyone know or sense my needs if I appeared not to need anything?"

Learning to express her needs in a healthy manner was up to Angie, not to some guy trying to read her mind.

"Lord knows they have enough trouble trying to figure out what THEY need," she laughed. "Some never have a clue about themselves, so they certainly can't second guess someone like me."

About a month before the divorce ended a 20-year marriage that included almost a two year separation, Angie found herself missing her soon-to-be-ex.

"It was more for companionship, for someone to talk to," she said. "It was more like being comfortable with an old habit, because in my notes regarding this feeling, I point out I do not 'want' him."

She also penned herself the question: "How long does it take from REjection to Ejection for another life?" She continued writing her thoughts as the marriage ended:

The void sometimes becomes a canyon
Although I'd never let you know
There were so many words, so many whys
Yet only sounds and no answers.
And 'because' echoes in the chasm
  am I stubborn?
  am I lonely?
  am I living in reality?
Quiet moments of joy and peace do come
And inside the answers quietly speak.
But days are long
  and nights are treasured.
Some day there'll be someone.

But for now, I hurt. Do you?
I realize how fragile I am
And I fear the edge of the canyon
And the rocks below if I fall.
God, grant me the Serenity,
  and acceptance
  and forgiveness
And the trust to take each day
  as a gift
  all wrapped up
Sometimes in brown paper with string,
But often with tinsel and bows.
Thank you for today's package – ME!

When All is Lost in the Process...

Connie's story leading to divorce is quite different from Angie's, except for the emotional pain which is the common denominator for all in this difficult process.

Given her background, her life was quite predictable. The first-born in an alcoholic family, Connie's earliest memory was that of her father trying to throw her baby sister out the window. Connie was only 2 years old, but from that instant when she froze in horror and her mother chased her from the room, she basically separated from everyone in the world.

"A part of me went into a glass cage," she said. "As the years went by the abuse got worse. Verbal assassination progressed to physical beatings and eventually incest."

At age 19 she was on her own, choosing not to move across country with the family. When she joined them a couple years later, she married the first man who offered an escape. She was not aware at the time that she was continuing the abuse. From the first day of marriage, her new husband's method of control was to belittle, demean and then demand.

"In that sense, my husband was my father, and when we had children, the pattern continued," she said. "My daughter was the first and she idolized her father. She became his little girl slave, with him mentally controlling her. I am not sure if he ever physically abused her, but she certainly attracted an abusive boyfriend later on."

Because her husband's father was a raging alcoholic, he never allowed alcohol in the house. With the mental control over the whole family, Connie said it was like walking on eggs.

"As time went on I discovered Valium. This comforted

me for years, allowing me to escape and detach from the reality of my surroundings," she said.

"My memory is that my father was a terrorist and my mother a Zombie. I have no idea if she was drinking or taking drugs, but she certainly escaped into her head. She just wasn't there."

By the time Connie hit her bottom, her daughter was 18 and had escaped the house. Her two sons were age 16 and 13. She entered a treatment program and was immediately banished from her family. It was as if one day she went to work, came back, the locks were changed and her things were on the porch.

"Emotionally, that's what happened," she said. "It broke my heart, but it didn't kill my spirit. It was an unmerciful thing, but I know now that complete deflation of ego was necessary."

She said she had always prided herself in being a good mother, only to find out 20 some years later that she was guilty of "emotional absence" from her family, the same way her mother wasn't there for her. Routine things got done, but she was unable to nurture.

As a functional alcoholic, Connie never lost a job, but the people close to her never received their full share because she "didn't have a clue on what to do or give."

She said as alcoholics, we are so "out of it" on how we behave and affect other people, so self-centered, that we can't possibly see ourselves as others perceive us.

When she couldn't return home after treatment, she had to find shelter and was referred to a halfway house – what a grounding in AA principles!

Doing the 12 Steps and meditating twice a day, having to take the responsibility of going out and getting a menial job to help pay her way and being responsible for herself in an adult way was all new territory.

While in the halfway house, a hurricane warning was in effect for the area, and everyone had to return to their respective homes until the storm passed.

"I went kicking and screaming and panicked. I couldn't stay in the halfway house. They didn't want me at home – what was I to do to stay sober?"

At home she was pounded by old behavior and her husband lashing out. The boys walked around silently looking at her as if to ask, "Who are you?" Connie doesn't blame them today, knowing their ignorance of the disease was compounded by their own inability to feel.

"The alcoholic is the natural scapegoat for blame in the family," she pointed out. Her husband wouldn't go to therapy but agreed to some Al-Anon meetings, after which he would berate and belittle her over her alcoholism.

"I received no credit for going through what I went through. He expected me to come home well, and well to him meant he could have complete control of me as he had before without the alcoholic outbursts of anger," she said. When old behavior stopped, when she came back with logic and not anger, he didn't know how to deal with it. He needed to keep pointing the finger. Therapy was suggested, but he left after two sessions. The therapist assured her that when he was ready he would return to therapy. It happened about seven years later, after the divorce, and after years of no communication. Even through therapy there was no communication. Connie believes that the family dysfunction was so broad that when he went with her to therapy, he couldn't cope.

A neighbor confided a while later that the night before Connie was due to come home from the halfway house, her husband and sons took a vote (her daughter was out drinking and drugging somewhere), which had to be unanimous on whether she should be let back in the house. She made it by only one vote. Two of the three didn't want her back.

Connie knew that to get well she would have to leave her family, to give up life as she knew it. She was not willing to sacrifice again. For the first time in her life she put herself first and has stayed there ever since, tending to her needs and her own happiness. The family left behind felt abandoned but also relieved. Her husband stopped going to Al-Anon.

Because her youngest son wanted to go with her when she left, she believes he's the one who voted in her favor.

"I told him I wasn't leaving because I didn't love him or want him, but so that I could survive and get well," she said. "I'm sure at 15 he still felt rejected, but it was the only thing I could do." Her oldest was 18 at the time, both boys well-conditioned by alcoholism.

The story of her daughter follows in another section of this book, but since leaving the marital home, Connie has had almost no contact with either of her sons. She's written long letters making amends and has talked to them on different occasions. There are no recriminations from them; they have both told her they love her, but have chosen not to maintain a relationship. Her ex-husband's influence was stronger over the years than the little nurturing she was able to give them earlier in life.

Connie didn't realize until therapy why she had so much resentment toward her mother. "She was physically present but never emotionally there for us. I was finally able to see that I was just like her, repeating the pattern with my children."

She feels her life really began at the age of 44 when she got sober because she didn't feel anything before then. She has forgiven herself and her family, including her mother, and today relies on her AA "family" for emotional guidance and assurance that she is "okay."

Affirmations

A year after Angie's divorce, she was encouraged to write some affirmations, reminders that would help her move on with her life. This is what she wrote at nine years sober:

I deserve someone who will celebrate life with me, someone who is positive, who can share on an intimate, personal level.

I deserve to be treated with respect, to be valued. I do NOT have to settle for anything less, for I am worthy of more.

I have had my trials, the dependency, the mental battering. I have had the negative, the oppressive, the arrogant.

I choose to live differently.

I choose to be me, to be the mother I want to be, to grow as my God wants me. I choose life, the pursuit of happiness and the chance to grow.

I am planting my garden, basking in the light and sinking roots into a new beginning. I want no weeds to interfere or strangle my convictions, no person to shadow the buds now forming.

I am free, I am deserving and I am terrific! Anyone who doesn't agree can bite the dust. Anyone who does – welcome!

Suggestions for going through divorce

❀ Attend at least one women's meeting of Alcoholics Anonymous each week. This is where you'll find women who have been through the same situation you are in.
❀ Be sure to have a sponsor to call at any time, particularly if you are still living with your partner.
❀ Go to some Al-Anon meetings if your partner is alcoholic, abusive or an addict.
❀ Work the steps with a sponsor, applying them to your situation.
❀ Try to recognize that neither person is entirely to blame...try to accept 50 percent of the responsibility, even if you don't believe you are to blame. It helps to relieve anger.
❀ Look to outside therapy, or to self-help groups on divorce, anger management or depression.
❀ Ask God to help you each day to make rational decisions.
❀ Ask God to help you with your response to abrasive or abusive comments from your partner.
❀ Remember: "Nothing changes, nothing changes." If you change, the situation changes.
❀ Because we are often very needy during a crisis such as divorce, and because we tend to repeat our patterns until they are broken, avoid any relationship with someone new until you are on your own and well. Chances are anyone who comes into your life at your most vulnerable point is also needy, a caretaker or a "fixer" in the guise of sympathy for your situation. Stick with the women, not the men, during a time of crisis.

Children

Children of alcoholics are given a tremendous burden, with possible damage in proportion to the severity of abuse and how long they have had to live in this condition. When a parent or parents get sober and begin to heal and recover, so do the children. Alcoholism is a family disease. Even if people are not alcoholic, if they live with the disease, they are affected, often in greater proportion than the alcoholic. Their lives revolve around and are dictated by the disease. If it is severe, they will avoid inviting friends to the house for fear the "elephant," that overwhelmingly huge problem in the house, might be seen. Children learn to stay out of the elephant's way and often retreat to the comfort of their room, to silence and their fantasies. They pretend that the elephant is not there. But it is so huge, so overwhelming, that eventually it "gets" them.

Angie posed the question: How do we, as newly recovering women, address the needs of our children while we are so desperate for answers ourselves?

"My children were a concern even in my drinking. When I went to treatment, I left a tape of me singing all their bedtime songs so they would have some continuity to their lives when I couldn't be there," she said, noting that even a "sick" parent is better than "no" parent to a child. She pointed out that children become accustomed to the mood swings, the parental arguing, verbal and even physical abuse. It becomes part of their daily routine, so when this is disrupted, even by recovery, they are at a loss. The elephant may be in another room, but it's still there.

"I was fortunate that my children were only 4 and 8 years old when I began my journey of sobriety, this total change of routine, personality and attitude," she said.

"While my son, the oldest, has recollection of bringing me beers in the backyard as I was sunning, there weren't deep, severe scars as a result of our drinking routine."

But they were still affected.

She remembered many times dinner had to wait when they were hungry because another drink was more important than eating. The children were often put to bed early (or sent to their rooms) because she and her husband were busy with their drinking and didn't want to bother interacting with them.

"I would feel guilt, shame, or despair looking at these beautiful children," she said, shaking her head as if to forget.

As Angie's drinking progressed, her parenting deteriorated, yet she said it was never really "that bad."

"They were fed, clothed, loved and cherished," she said. "Because my 'bottom' was only about six months, most of the damage was done in that time. Booze robbed them of quality time from me, mostly in the evening, as that is when I drank. They were always on time for school, help was usually there for homework, and to the outside world, we were a wonderful little family."

But once the elephant moved in permanently instead of visiting occasionally, her little family began to crumble under its heavy feet.

"In truth, I was gripped with fear of hurting these precious children, of damaging them forever," she said. "I thank God I was led to sobriety before destroying them."

Angie laughed as she recalled how their little cockerpoo dog began doing his business in the house as their drinking progressed.

"When we got sober, his bad habits stopped. Alcoholism IS a family disease!"

Once she returned from treatment (her ex-husband had

told them Mommy wouldn't be crazy anymore) she was able to introduce the 12 Steps into her daily life, which of course, included parenting. Angie said she'll never forget the first time she heard her daughter, at age 5, saying out loud, "God grant me the serenity...!" Or the time they had an upset and her son asked, "Does this mean I have to do a Step Ten?"

"I tried to be as honest and outspoken about my recovery as I could with the children, explaining how so many years of drinking had turned me into someone I didn't want to be," said Angie. "By not drinking, the healing began."

With a parent going to a meeting every night of the week, the children not only experienced recovery, but became involved in 12-step work and visually were able to see how "bad" it "could" have gotten.

One incident that always comes to Angie's mind involves 12-stepping a Swedish girl. In the early days of her sobriety, 12-step work was still being done, where two alcoholics would actually go to a person's house to help.

"In this particular case, my friend and I brought this young woman back to my house because her partner was physically abusive and she needed to get out of her particular situation immediately, at least for a few hours, to decide what she was going to do," Angie recalled. "She was a mess. Her makeup was smeared, her hair uncombed, her eyes hollow, her clothes wrinkled and spotted. My daughter, about age 6 at the time, went up to her, patted her on the back and said, 'That's okay. You'll get better. My Mommy was MUCH worse than you!' So much for MY perception of how my children viewed me at the end of my drinking!"

Alcoholics became part of their everyday family life, and Angie and her husband often talked openly to the children about recovery.

"Basically, the elephant was invited to eat at the table,

to become part of the family," she said. "By taming it with knowledge, compassion, understanding and change, it was no longer the frightening beast."

Because Angie feels so strongly in family recovery as a result of parents being sober, she made a special request of her home AA group when she reached the five-year mark. In addition to her celebrating, she presented each of her children with a five-year medallion.

"There wasn't a dry eye in the room," she smiled. "I still get emotional when I remember that night."

When her son was 13 years old, he began attending an Alateen meeting where she went to a step meeting.

"One Tuesday driving home, he told me to congratulate him. I asked why? He announced he had just received his year medallion. I couldn't believe how fast the year had gone by and how much progress had been made. I was so happy for him."

While this was the last meeting he attended (it was no longer a cool thing to do) he nonetheless got his own recovery foundation. Angie said another reason for not returning was to avoid some members who were drinking and drugging, a decision based on what was good for him personally.

In the first few years of sobriety Angie also attended Al-Anon meetings.

"I needed tools on how to live with an alcoholic, even if he was in recovery," she said, adding that she still goes occasionally for a "booster shot" to deal with the alcoholic personalities in her life.

Cunning, Baffling, Powerful – and Patient!

Judy had a different situation with her children. She never started drinking until she was 39, "a divorced grownup."

Angie first met Judy when she was newly sober.

"I was invited to her 40th birthday party and can remember feeling out of place as a sober person. Everyone was drinking and having a good time. I watched Judy get thrown into the swimming pool fully clothed, followed by many of the guests. I knew it was not a healthy place for me to be and left."

She knew Judy understood because Angie had previously shared with her that she was an alcoholic and couldn't drink, and that she had gone to AA. Over the years they remained friends but Angie avoided parties where everyone was drinking.

"I watched Judy's career advance and did not see her often enough to watch the progression of her disease," she said.

By the time Judy was 49, her alcoholism was full-blown. Her children were in college and couldn't wait to get out of the house when home on vacation. They no longer knew their mother and were facing their own problems created by living in a dysfunctional family.

How did Judy get to this point in only 10 years of drinking?

She said she had tried drinking earlier in life, and each time she drank she got "wasted and sick." She can remember drinking with a friend in high school when the parents were out of town, climbing a tree and not being able to get down. On festive occasions, she'd have a sip of whatever was being offered, but she didn't "drink" until her brother got married in 1977. She was with friends and lots of family members. The bartender asked her what she wanted to drink, and out of the blue, she said "Scotch." He gave her a large glass, then another...Judy said she "felt fine. I could finally drink without getting sick." Reflecting back years later, she pointed out that alcoholism was progressing from her high school days on, whether or not she drank in the interim. By the time she ordered the Scotch, she was already a "pickle," referring to the story of how everyone starts life as a "cucumber" with some becoming "pickles" along the way. A "pickle" can never again be a "cucumber."

A few months later her sister died in a motorcycle accident. Judy was devastated. They had been extremely close, almost like twins. Their children were about the same age, and when her sister died, she found herself a mother of four instead of two children, ranging in age from 6 to 9 years old. Six weeks later she got married, as previously planned. She now had a new husband and four children. She turned to alcohol to relieve the pain and cope with all the changes, and escaped into a new career, getting her pilot's license in 1978.

"I had two loves – my kids and flying," she said. "I also had a love for drinking, but I didn't mix the two. That was a built-in control, an absolute law for me. When I was in an airplane I couldn't think of my sister's death, all the kids, my marriage or other problems in the family."

When her mother was dying of cancer, she and her husband moved to Florida. Her children stayed in the northeast with their father, and her nieces with their father. Judy devoted herself to helping her mother and flying, achieving all the ratings of a professional pilot. But her increased drinking put pressure not only on her flying career, but on her deteriorating marriage.

In a period of only six weeks she was divorced, her

mother died and the children, now college age, moved back to a home and parent they hardly recognized. It was total chaos. In the next few years her daughter developed an eating disorder and her son chalked up a number of tickets for operating a motorcycle under the influence when he went off to college. He also suffered from a chronic stomach disorder that had to be treated with prescription narcotics.

In 1987, when the children were 19 and 21 years of age, Judy had been drinking for ten years – ten years that made up for all the years that she didn't drink from high school to when she had that Scotch.

"I started making dinner the night before they were going back to college and, of course, was drinking while preparing the food. I knew I had to fly a small charter plane the next morning. I also realized I was too drunk to sit down to dinner with them," she said. "They were disgusted with me. I went to my room, then took some of my son's pills to really punish myself. I made my usual pleas to God to help me out of this one and passed out."

When she awoke at 6 o'clock the next morning to fly, everything had changed. She knew it was too early to call the friend she knew could help. She waited until 7 a.m. to call Angie, who was surprised to hear from Judy at that hour but happy that she wanted to go to a meeting.

"I can remember feeling an emotional high all day, praying that her flight would be safe. I was in awe that God had chosen me to take Judy to her first meeting of Alcoholics Anonymous," said Angie. "I had no idea of the power my sobriety had had on my dear friend over all those years."

Judy's daughter was thrilled she was sober, because she was already experiencing recovery from an eating disorder. Her son was less enthusiastic, not really knowing or understanding this new mother.

"I drank from the time he was 9 years old to 19," said Judy. "Those were important, difficult years for him. After I got sober he would speak to me, but there was no real connection. It was like a veil over the relationship. I couldn't get through to him, even though he had chosen to become a professional pilot and we had much in common."

When she was eight years sober, they flew together on a trip.

"He was arguing with me about something," Judy said. "I calmly told him that we can disagree about anything we want, that we can just love each other or even just like each other, but we don't have to agree."

That was the beginning of change, for him to open up to her, to be honest about what he was feeling and thinking.

By the time she was 14 years sober, Judy was the first to be called when he passed an important flight check ride, even before his wife.

"This was a total miracle," said Judy. "I never thought that veil would be lifted. I certainly didn't think my son would become one of my best friends. It happened early on with my daughter, so this breakthrough was special. We're finally the family we've always wanted to be, even though we are all adults living in different parts of the country. We have love, understanding and we truly value one another. This is possible only because I got sober."

She pointed out that it was the consistency of her program a day at a time that brought peace to the chaos in the family.

Both her adult children have shared that they blamed themselves for their mother's condition, thinking they were at fault.

"They didn't know what to do with this mom who was

supposed to back them and help them," she said. "They knew that something was terribly wrong, yet they were loyal to me even when they were repulsed by the creature passed out on the kitchen floor. They just stuffed it away, as do all family members of the alcoholic."

The important point today is that her children feel comfortable talking and sharing about both the good and difficult times, thankful that their mother is there for them – a sober grownup.

The Daughter's Point of View

Camie, Judy's daughter, has memories of a normal childhood in the northeast. Her mother was the best, always there for her children, nurturing them, caring for them, proud of them, shielding them from discomforts and events leading to the deterioration of the marriage.

It all changed when Camie entered her teen years. Her parents divorced and she moved to Florida with her mother. She only stayed for about six months, then went back to live with her father to finish high school in more familiar, comfortable surroundings. She hated Florida and just couldn't adjust to the new lifestyle and the changes taking place with her mother. During her many vacation visits, exposure to her mother's drinking was unavoidable. With her mother's love affair with booze and a new boyfriend who also drank and a younger brother who was now experimenting with drugs, Camie felt alone. She craved attention.

"I remember feeling frustrated about mom's drinking and how I couldn't do anything about it," she said.

If drugs were brought into the house, everyone did them. Her brother's anger increased as his addiction escalated and Camie was swept along in all the uncertainty, unpredictability and insanity of a family on a too-fast track.

"It was almost as if we were all just waiting for something to happen," she said.

For Camie, escape was not only into drinking and drugs, but she became obsessed with her weight. She would diet, become thin and get the approval of peers. The obsession grew. Before long she was throwing up on a regular basis, a victim of bulimia. While her body deteriorated, her sadness was overwhelming.

"I hung out with all the wrong people who were like

me," she said. "It seemed I was out of touch with everything from the time my parents divorced and mom started drinking, but I believe it would have all happened anyway."

Her mother, still in the throes of alcoholism, began "catching" Camie vomiting on several occasions. She knew something was terribly wrong but until Camie was in a terrible car crash and the crisis reached another level, couldn't get her help. Even drowning in her own addiction, Judy wanted to be a good mother, to still do what was right for her precious children. She insisted Camie see a counselor, but the emphasis was on drinking and drugs and Camie feels the counselor "never got it." Bulimia was still in the closet.

By the time she was a freshman in college, she admitted her terrible secret. Her mother was still drinking, but managed to get Camie into a day treatment program.

"Mom was always there physically, but was not emotionally available when she was drinking," she said. "I would call her and know something was terribly wrong. Her speech would be slurred and she wouldn't remember what I told her. It was terrible. I felt I had lost her."

Following day treatment, Camie went to a therapist who worked with the entire family, including her father, but all the addictions continued, including bulimia. When Judy feared for her daughter's life, she gave her an ultimatum. Either she "pull it together on her own" or get treatment. Camie knew it was impossible to stop on her own, so agreed to a residential program at a respected eating disorder treatment center.

That was the year that everything changed again. Her mother was given the gift of sobriety.

"Mom was so happy with her new life and all that she was learning in AA," said Camie. "She became the mother of my childhood again, nurturing, attentive, caring, yet it was so different. She visited me often, flying across country, and kept talking about the program, the 12 steps, how I could use a tree as my higher power if I couldn't believe in God. She was on a mission to save her children, to be there for us even though we were now both adults. We became a family again, with everyone concerned about one another, pulling together to be free of addiction."

While drinking was an issue, Camie admits her eating disorder was her "bottom." She tried several 12 Step programs, but she has decided her best recovery is in Alcoholics Anonymous.

Now, several years later, the whole family is still sober, free of drugs and Camie has conquered bulimia, but it's a day at a time, with everyone working their individual programs. Camie is married and a massage therapist. Her brother is a professional pilot, following in his mother's footsteps, and Judy is enjoying retirement, married to another recovering retired airline pilot. AA not only saved each one individually, but the family as a whole. They are all fun people to be around – definitely happy and free of addictions that almost killed the entire family.

Suggestions for helping your children

- ✿ Be honest about your recovery. Children see life situations on television every day. No matter how young, they will understand if you are honest.
- ✿ If you have pre-teens or teens, provide them with literature that is available for their age group on alcoholism. If possible, have them attend Alateen meetings.
- ✿ Children of alcoholics have been through a lot of

emotional turmoil. Give them more hugs than before, and tell them, as well as show them, how much you love them, no matter what has taken place in the past.
- Ask your children to help in your recovery. Allow them to remind you if they see old behavior that frightens them, that it's okay for them to be honest about their feelings.
- Introduce them to some of the program slogans: Easy Does It, One Day At A Time, etc.
- Share the Serenity Prayer, and explain acceptance of a situation if there is nothing else that can be done.
- Talk about change, particularly if one parent is not in recovery, that we can only change ourselves, not another person.
- Do not allow your children to manipulate you like in the past when you were drinking. Say "no" and mean it with love. You do not have to explain why.
- Remember that just as it took years to come into the program and get sober, it may take time for children to accept the new parent in their lives. Be patient and be consistent. No matter what their age, it's possible to restore a relationship.
- Finally, be aware of what's going on in the family. If there is even a hint that your children are drinking or experimenting with drugs, or show unusual weight loss, don't wait until there is a crisis – get help for them as soon as possible, even though they will deny there is a problem.

Death

This is a tough subject for any alcoholic, and Angie had a great deal to share on the subject. In reality, many of us "died" at the end of our drinking, with true life beginning only in sobriety. Old ideas, old habits, old friends...all let go so a new life could thrive.

She has always been drawn to the Prayer of St. Francis which is also referenced in Step Eleven in the "12 and 12" of AA: that it is in "dying that we are born to eternal life."

My 'death' was the beginning of recovery and my acceptance of my disease. It became the springboard to a new way of life that encompasses all.

Angie's writings March 1983

With the new sense of awareness, compassion and feeling that comes with sobriety, the death of a family member, a close friend or someone in the program becomes a totally different experience. In the past, funerals usually meant drinking, numbing feelings, masking our inability for true compassion. Now that we are able to truly feel sorrow, we can be emotionally available for family and friends in their time of grief. Words have meaning.

Often loved ones died before we got sober, before we could make our amends. For Angie, her father's death was a milestone in her life because it led her to enter treatment and get sober.

"When he died, I was still drinking. I couldn't get in touch with my feelings. I couldn't be the support I should have been to my mother and siblings," she said. "It wasn't until treatment over a month later that I could deal with his death, cry 'real' tears, experience sorrow as I had never done before."

Through the help of a counselor and grief therapy, she was able to see how she was carrying through his last wishes by getting sober. Now, after so many years in the program, her amends have been made. How she lives today is important.

"Since coming into the program, I have lost many women who were influential in my sobriety: Eve M., who died with 50-some years and who gave the final address at the international convention in Seattle in 1990; Eleanor with 40-some years; Ruth H. and Alberta, who gave so much service to recovering alcoholics. So many friends in the program who died sober – Bill and Peggy K, Christine, Jim M.

And then there's Richard. Angie sat silently for a few minutes, took a deep breath, and said, "This won't be easy, even after so many years. I still feel Richard is with me today, even though someone else is in my life and so many circumstances have changed."

A Love Story

Angie had been divorced about two years when Richard came into her life. He had four years of sobriety and she was approaching the nine-year mark. She would catch him staring at her during meetings, smiling when she was talking with people after.

"He wasn't that physically attractive: rather skinny, balding with large glasses that dominated and pointed chin," she said. "It was the softness in his eyes, the gentle tone of his voice, a glimpse of his spirit, that drew me to him."

Before they met, he was already planning to move to another part of the state, so Angie was extremely cautious on getting involved. She said he was more than a perfect gentleman.

The relationship began by writing letters and cards and sitting for hours at all-night restaurants following AA meetings.

"We never talked on the phone because he was separated from his wife but still living in the same house, waiting for it to be sold and the divorce to be final," she said. "I had not intended to get involved with someone who was still married and who had not lived on his own, and I certainly didn't want a 'rebound' from a previous relationship."

His friends confirmed what he had told her, that he and his wife shared space since sobriety, but not a home. He moved to the house where his office was located, converting an office to a bedroom. They could finally talk on the phone, but the letters and cards continued.

Angie said his refuge was the seventh floor of the city library. There he would read poetry, his favorite being Rumi, write, read/study Emmett Fox's *Sermon on the Mount*, and another favorite author, Scott Peck. He often quoted from

What Return Can I Make and *The Road Less Traveled*.

Richard was on a spiritual quest, a cancer survivor who was given a chance for new life in sobriety, who put his spiritual development ahead of everything else in his life.

He told Angie he hadn't planned on falling in love, but wrote, "Here was the positive to match the negative, matching so closely it became almost frightening at the clarity with which God can synthesize."

"Intellectually we may have been a good match, but he was physically distant, introspective in his own spiritual development, and often quiet, frustrating me to no end," said Angie. "I was much more outgoing."

She said they talked about patience, about the avoidance of "instant gratification." At times she wanted to run, to end the relationship.

"It wasn't at all what I thought I wanted, and certainly did not follow what happened in the past. He seemed almost weird," she said, "yet I couldn't turn away. Something exciting was developing. I joked that maybe our spirits were having some fun."

As usual, she turned to her writing to express her feelings. At this point she had no idea where God was taking the relationship or how the "big picture" would be revealed.

I slid down gently, grasping the reins of reality.
It happened so quietly, so sweetly,
But the pain was there.
Quiet, clear, the mirror shattered.

I felt cheated but whole.
I reached for old tapes and they were gone.
You gave me new ones.
Real ones.

Something to soothe the spirit.
Kyrie eleison.
You never touched me but reached my soul,
That indefinable someplace more real than flesh.
Then you let go
And the invisible crashed.
Praise Him with clanging cymbals.
I was too trusting to ask,
Too new to the game, too raw from the last round.
That wound bears a scar.
This one did not bleed.
It will heal.
I'll sing His praise and carry on.
And time will treasure the moments with you.
Without you.

Sadness overwhelmed me and I dissolved it with tears.
I mourned what might not be, even tomorrow.
And I know what I deserve.

I deserve moonlit walks on the ocean
And Serene island nights.
I deserve to celebrate life
With someone holding my hand.
Who can claim me and possess me
Without ownership.
Someone who expects nothing
And accepts everything,
Who gives everything
And demands nothing.
Someone who can live and be loved
In every sense, on every level,
In any place, for all time.

That person is there, somewhere,
And you may be in-between, somewhere.
Here, but not there.
And yet not all here.
Even when you're with me I am often alone.
So be it.
Kyrie eleison!
P.S.
Thank you for this burst of thoughts,
And for being you.
We have both gained something
If not everything.
Cheers to life's ups and downs,
Ins and outs and wonderful nows.
Take care,
God bless!
***

These lessons are a bitch.

Angie's writings

After his divorce they became closer, sharing on a more intimate, yet spiritual level.

"I had never knelt and prayed with a man before, but this became part of our routine," she said. "We remained close to friends in the program and our sponsors, unlike many couples who, once they find each other, become consumed with one another to the exclusion of everyone else.

It was definitely not a normal situation, and as time went on, he met her mother and siblings and they began making plans for a life together with everyone's blessing. Richard commented how he had never felt so welcomed as in Angie's mother's house.

By Christmas of 1988 it was almost a year that they had

been seeing each other, living separately but often traveling together and taking weekends to different parts of the state. Angie's daughter, now in high school, was very comfortable with Richard and they did family things together. Her son, on the other hand, did not like the idea of another man in his mother's life, and when Angie informed him she would be marrying Richard, her son chose to live with his father after returning from boarding school.

"This deeply saddened me and I cried often, as my son is precious to me. But I was not going to be held hostage, to let him rule the house when it was still my house," she said. "I told him I was building a new life, that it could include him, but I know he felt threatened. It was a typical male knee-jerk reaction, but since his father lived only minutes away, I was still nearby and participated in his upbringing and decisions for his future. I will admit, though, that this was a sad time for me: on the one hand I had love I had never experienced in my life and on the other I felt I had lost my son. But I knew it was not a fair choice: it wasn't which apple do you want...it was you can have this or nothing at all."

Richard was also saddened by her son's decision as he really wanted to get to know this person who was so much a part of Angie, particularly since her daughter so readily accepted him.

"We prayed a lot for my son, and also for my ex-husband," said Angie. "I was still carrying a tremendous amount of anger over the separation, divorce, settlement and his lack of involvement with the children."

Through prayer, just as it talks about in "Freedom from Bondage," the last chapter in the "Big Book," she was able to let go of the anger, to forgive him, and to appreciate that her son at least had a father he could turn to. But it was rough times for all of them, especially when Richard said he was having difficulty swallowing, that he was looking forward to his annual checkup to see if there were any more problems arising from his cancer, originally in the right jaw, then in the salivary glands.

"He always had to have water by his side, but after five years of good checkups, he wasn't particularly worried," she said, reflecting back on how positive they both were at the time.

In January they traveled to Denver so one of his best friends could meet Angie.

"We had a wonderful week in the mountains," she reflected. "I went ice skating for the first time since I was a kid and we really enjoyed ourselves. On the return, we stopped in Houston for his checkup. He was in the hospital for several hours, and when he came out, he told me we'd know the outcome of the tests in a few days. But he was very quiet and introspective. We didn't hear our flight announced, missed it, and had to fly to another city and rent a car to get home that night. When we called my daughter to tell her the new arrival time, she was distraught. The parakeet Richard had given her, Figgy, had died that day. Richard's comment was that he wasn't surprised. I asked him why he said that and he just shrugged. No comment, no emotion. I thought it very strange."

In the next few days she kept asking if he'd found out about the tests and he kept telling her he didn't know as yet, but not to worry.

"When almost a month passed and he still had not heard from the doctors or hospital, I began to get suspicious." she said. "Richard was sleeping more, drinking more liquid, talking less because of the dryness in his mouth and pouring himself into his work, studying for a difficult state exam."

They were spending a lot of quality time with each other, but because they weren't living together, there was a lot of commuting across town, attending several AA meetings a week, working with sponsees and also with their sponsors on a personal level.

"We wanted to make sure it was in God's plan for both of us to be together," she said. "He took the state exam he had been studying so hard for on February 17 and 18 and to celebrate, we spent the weekend away from home, returning Sunday night. He was quiet, but I chalked it up to the stress and aftermath of taking the exam."

Angie never expected what happened next.

On Monday, when she couldn't reach Richard by phone, Angie spoke to the office secretary who said he was sleeping and not working. He had told her not to disturb him. Angie met him at the usual Monday night AA meeting they both attended, arriving at different times and ending up at different ends of the room. About half-way through the meeting Angie noticed Richard was gone. No explanation, no way of knowing what had happened.

"After the meeting I went to his home/office. He was already in bed." Angie put her head in her hands, holding back tears. "He told me he was dying, that the cancer was in his throat, that it was inoperable and that he maybe had six to twelve months to live. He had known since the day he walked out of the hospital in Denver but wanted to spare me as long as possible. The emotional pain was so excruciating I felt someone had physically shot me. It was one of our most horrifying yet close moments together. I cried, and as the tears poured out, I felt my insides hollowing, with nothing to fill the pain. It was so terrible that I could not even stay with him. Fear and panic left me devastated. I drove home blinded by tears and called my family...my mother, my brothers one by one...it was midnight before I went to bed and cried myself to sleep. The miracle is that I never once thought of drinking."

By the next night Richard was very ill, delirious and talking nonsense. Angie took him to the emergency room where his doctor met them.

"I found out Richard's silence was also due to drugs he was already taking to ease his pain," she said.

He never again slept at his office room. If they were only to have a few months together, they were going to make the most of it. Richard talked about going to a VA hospital to "spare" Angie.

"I told him he didn't have that right, that I was going to help him through to the end," she said.

His journey to death included daily prayer and meditation, AA meetings brought to the home, and a constant parade of sponsees, sponsors, AA friends and family.

Through prayer, understanding and an unbelievable love for each other and God, they were carried along the path.

"Never did our faith in each other or God waiver," she said. "Our AA program helped us through each day to whatever lay ahead."

A quiet acceptance and peace developed, knowing that there was no "turning back," that they had absolutely no control over the course or direction of Richard's journey.

"Instead of fighting the situation, we prepared for it. I pulled out the scrubby ixora hedge and we planted flowers and beautiful greens so he could see the waterway from the bed," she said. "He painstakingly built trellises so that bouganvillea could climb overhead. The bird feeder was filled with seed each day, and a pair of cardinals became daily visitors, coming ever closer to him as he meditated."

One day Richard looked out from his bed and said, "This is a nice place to die."

He began spending longer hours each day meditating on the back porch, with friends visiting more and more to listen to his quiet wisdom, to hear whatever they could to help their own journey, sensing that he was totally connected to his God and that he was at peace even with all the pain. Angie said Richard never complained, only "reported" his feelings, his concern for her and her children.

"He drew up his will and made his own funeral arrangements," she said, and his 83-year-old mother came to live with us for a couple of weeks. She was a difficult, self-centered woman. Richard had warned me about her, but I felt it important that she be with her son."

There were several difficulties to overcome during Richard's convalescence. Because his throat was increasingly sore, Richard explored foods that he could swallow but still keep his taste buds happy...bleu cheese, caviar and cream cheeses.

"What feasts he prepared for the two of us on thin crackers!" she smiled. "Every night we prayed together, held each other, and loved each other in the best way we possibly could. My sole purpose was to ease his pain, to help him in any way I could, even though I felt helpless so many times, the only thing I could do was pray and ask God for relief of pain for him."

Angie began to truly sense what one day at a time was. At one point, one of the many AA visitors talked about doing something in August. She thought, "August... August."

"It was inconceivable for me to think beyond the moment, beyond the day," she said. "To me, August was an eternity, just as the next day was. It became more and more difficult to concentrate on my work except on a day-to-day basis, and to approach each day in terms of food, planning, school, and work as the only day I had."

They saw little miracles taking place. One of his sponsees, plagued with depression, began pulling out of it. Another who had called himself an atheist physically saw the power of God working in Richard's life and "came to believe." Old friends came to visit, not recognizing the person they still remembered from drinking days.

"On Sunday, April 18, he wanted to talk with me and my daughter," said Angie. "He told us he didn't think he had much longer. My daughter had made a bracelet of colorful string which she put on his wrist for good luck. We were both in denial of his words. He didn't look that bad, but he insisted the end was at hand."

Monday night he lapsed into a coma and hospice went on 24 hour duty, with a nurse in the home every minute to help.

"Prior to that, hospice was on call if I needed them and came regularly to administer his meds," said Angie. "One of the nurses that morning commented how calm and accepting everyone was. There were always many AAs in the house and she began to pick up on these 'different' people. When she found out none of us drank, she talked about her husband who had just entered treatment. She had no concept of alcoholism, but by the end of the day found herself loved by AAs and Al-anons, with lots of hope for her family. Coincidental? I don't think so. God chose her to be with us that day."

Tuesday night Richard was still in a coma and on Wednesday, at 11:15 a.m., he took his last breath.

"Everyone dear to him was at his side, including my daughter, who refused to go to school because she wanted to be with him," she said.

The promised six to twelve months was less than three.

Brandy, Angie's little dog, had been by Richard's side every day. After he died, she somehow was still in the room when the funeral people came.

"They let her out and she tore through the house making the most horrible sounds and acting like she wanted to bite everyone in the house," said Angie. "This went on for at least 15 minutes, startling all of us. Even Brandy had to express her grief."

Right after Richard died, Angie felt compelled to put on Vivaldi.

"Somehow his favorite CD was in the player and as the music began, I felt a sensation that I was 'launching' his soul," she said, reflecting. "For a moment, I felt total peace. Then indescribable grief set in and I needed every person in the room to help me through my agony. When my father had died, I went right to the bottle. Now, with the love of my life gone forever, drinking was not even a distant thought."

There were so many incidents, so many happenings, so many feelings to deal with in the course of Richard's death.

"I've only touched on part of this long two-month journey," said Angie. "God only gave us 14 months together, and the only two that we actually lived together focused on his impending death."

At his funeral, packed with AAs and family, Angie played the guitar and sang a spiritual song that was one of his favorites, that gave him strength in the dying process.

"No one knows how I managed to get through the entire song, but I did because it was the right thing to do, the last tribute I could make to this wonderful, inspirational, spiritual man who shared such a brief time in my own journey," she said. "I know today that I was put in his life to help him die. He was put in my life to help me live."

A Child's Suicide

Probably the worst "death" one can experience is the suicide of a child, no matter what age that offspring may be. For Connie it was a devastating incident that occurred when she was 16 months sober. Twenty years later the pain, the remembrance, the reality is still tangible. It never leaves her. Every birthday, every anniversary of "the day," is a reminder.

She said the grieving process was tremendous. She experienced guilt, shame, helplessness, anger, abandonment and isolation from the rest of the world.

"I got mad at God. How could He allow this to happen?"

She knows now that because of her own addictions, she couldn't see the signs in her daughter. Looking back, she recalls Barbara being resentful as early as the age of three when her new baby brother was born. When she was five years old and the second brother came home, she told her mother she wanted to be an only child. Connie believes her "walls" of anger went up at this early age, with Barbara wrapping her father around her little finger. She never saw any signs of alcohol or drugs until her daughter was 16 years old. She was drinking beer and smoking pot, but Connie chalked it up to normal kid behavior – she was just trying it out.

"In reality, I went into denial about what she was doing because I was in denial about my own situation," she said. Even when Barbara got kicked off the swim team when she was 17 years old, Connie couldn't read the signs. Barbara moved in with her abusive boyfriend. Connie's husband never said much about anything except to blame her if something went wrong – "You take care of it," he'd say.

"I couldn't take care of myself. How could I take care

of anyone else?" she asked.

After Connie got sober, Barbara came to see her at work one day when she was 19 years old. She wanted to borrow money and Connie asked her what for. She told her "lunch." So she said, "Why don't I take you to lunch?" she asked, admitting that she suspected Barbara wanted money for drugs. She gave her $10 when they parted. It wasn't until later that she discovered her husband had been giving Barbara money all along, which most likely paid for her drugs.

One day she was on the phone with Barbara giving her a dose of "tough love" she had learned about in treatment. In the background she heard a loud bang. She asked if her boyfriend was shooting at her because Connie knew the boyfriend dealt in stolen guns and dope. She asked Barbara if she wanted to come home and she said yes, but that her boyfriend wouldn't let her. Connie said, "Put him on the phone," and told him to let her go. Barbara came home, but then went back without any explanation. Connie found out later from some young people she met in AA that, more than likely, Barbara needed a fix and couldn't get it in the home because her mother was sober. Every time Connie asked if she was using Barbara said no, but Connie knew the truth.

"I told her I could help, that I could put her in touch with other people her age." She told her she couldn't stay in the family house but that she would find a place where Barbara would be safe. The boyfriend had threatened to kill her, so Connie took Barbara to the state mental hospital. She was then referred to Women in Distress, an outstanding facility that has sheltered more than 250,000 women and children since its founding by the late Edee Greene in 1974.

Barbara only stayed in the shelter for five weeks before

leaving and returning to the boyfriend, who had found out where she was. Years later, Barbara's counselor confided that the reason she went back was that he threatened to kill not only her, but her mother, father and two brothers. Connie heard nothing from Barbara until six months later when she came by to say hello. She was on crutches, and told Connie she was much better. Connie gave her a hug and could feel her ribs in the back. I thought, "Where's Barbara? Where's my daughter?" She was a skeleton, only a shell of a 20-year old woman.

Some time later, Connie answered the phone after returning from a Sunday night AA meeting. Someone was screaming for her to get to such-and-such address because Barbara had just blown her head off.

I said, "Thank you for letting me know this happened, but I don't need to have that as my last memory of her." She asked if someone had identified her, the answer was yes, and Connie replied, "Then there's no need for me to be there."

Connie called her AA sponsor, who picked her up and drove her around for hours while Connie cried, talked, screamed and went through the anguish any mother would over the tragic, horrible loss of her daughter. But she also thanked God for letting it happen at this time in her sobriety when she had a support system in place that enabled her to handle it.

Connie said Barbara was sitting on a huge bag of Qualudes when she put the .45 cal. to her head.

It took only four years from the time Barbara started drinking and drugging until her suicide. She was a little person, and alcohol and drugs destroyed her mind, body and spirit. A minister later explained to Connie that when she felt Barbara's ribs during the hug that she was already spiritually dead. He eased her guilt about taking her to the hospital, reassuring her that it was the right thing to do, that she could not have brought her home. Connie knew she was unable to keep Barbara sheltered and safe from drugs, alcohol and the abusive boyfriend.

The minister also told her that God let Barbara go so she could be free, and that when it was her turn to go she would see her again on the other side.

"I know she's with me today, she's just not physically on this planet," said Connie. "Spiritually we are connected through the God of my understanding even though her body is dead."

Following Barbara's death, the boyfriend called and said he wanted the body back to give her a Catholic funeral.

"I asked if they were married and he said no. I said, then the body belongs to the family." He threatened to kill the whole family, and while Connie kept him on the phone, told her husband what the boyfriend said. The husband then said he'd get a gun and stop him.

"I thought this was not the time to play John Wayne, and sent the boys to get the cop who lived across the street."

She kept the boyfriend on the phone long enough for the policeman to hear the threats. An all-points bulletin was put out and three area police departments began searching for him to Baker Act him. Connie remembers standing with her fists up to heaven screaming, "It's enough! Stop it NOW!" He was picked up within hours and locked up. When they found him he had a loaded gun and was heading towards Connie's home.

The night before the funeral, the hospital called to ask if they could let the boyfriend out a day early so he could go to Barbara's funeral. Connie said absolutely not, but when they called back her husband said, "certainly," that he could say goodbye to Barbara, but not during the funeral. He didn't tell Connie he countered her decision, but Connie never saw the boyfriend. "Apparently the police found stolen guns and drugs and put him in jail for six months, but he still threatened to kill us when he got out," she said. "Thank God we never heard from him again. If there is mercy, perhaps he is either dead or in jail."

The morning after Barbara died, Connie went to a ten o'clock AA meeting. Her husband was incensed that she was going to a meeting right after her daughter died. She told him that's where she belonged. She felt sick physically, as if she had pneumonia, but when she visited the doctor he told her no, it wasn't pneumonia, it was grief. He offered her drugs, a "fix," to feel better. She declined, saying she didn't need it and went to another AA meeting.

Connie said that two nights after Barbara died, she saw her face in a bright light. "She smiled at me with such sweetness and love. I never recalled her that way and I knew she was blissfully happy with God. The expression was incredible. It was like she knew everything."

When she told the minister about this he said, "Wow! They usually don't get to the other side that quickly!" He attributed it to the drugs having destroyed her so God took her. He told her others have tried to commit suicide, have grossly injured themselves and lived. God let Barbara die because she could not accomplish spiritual goals while locked in her addiction.

In retrospect, Connie feels that her return to the family home after the halfway house was part of God's plan. She tried three separate times while at the halfway house to find another living situation so she wouldn't have to return home. Each one fell through.

"Then one day I was standing at the sign-out sheet to

go to work when I got a feeling that a big hand was in the middle of my back. It seemed to shove me, and at the same time I got the thought to go home."

Her minister later told her she was supposed to be there when the phone call came about Barbara's suicide. She had to go home, to try and intervene, to help her and to be there, to get her to a safe place. She remembers having to fight with her husband and two sons, to stand fast that Barbara was an active druggie living with someone who deals and steals guns, that it was dangerous to have her in the house. It seemed like she was the only one with common sense or, as Connie translates it, a program for dealing with life situations.

"I couldn't be in denial anymore. I woke up in sobriety like someone threw a pail of cold water in my face."

Connie attended two meetings a day for about six months after Barbara's death.

"The women held me, listened to me, comforted me and gave me the strength I needed," she said. "Then one day it was like someone lifted a blanket off my head. It was over. That initial grief period lasted six months."

She could take a deep breath again and feel the air coming into her body. The worst was over, although she still has thoughts on whether she could have done something better or different. It's then that she uses her AA tools again, and again, and again. She believes everything that happened was necessary.

Connie initially thought about Barbara every day, then from time to time, especially on her birthday or the day she died. Today she is still sad, but not "hooked into it." There is relief in knowing it was Barbara's choice, her destiny, even though she still misses what they might have had if drugs and alcohol had not robbed them both of the relationship.

This is the first time Connie has been able to share the full story of Barbara's death and the abusive boyfriend. She pointed out that just as drugs and alcohol aren't good for us, we also choose people who aren't good for us. She hopes her daughter's story will help another mother, daughter or family.

Suggestions for dealing with death

- ❁ If a loved one is dying and you are the caregiver, share the difficulties with a friend or another family member. Be honest with how YOU feel. Being honest about your own needs, feelings and desires will help the loved one.
- ❁ If you are having trouble getting to meetings because you don't want to leave that person, invite your home group to meet in your home, or ask that someone give of their time so you can get to a meeting. You'll be surprised how many people want to do service if they have the opportunity.
- ❁ Stay close to a sponsor, letting her know what you're feeling.
- ❁ Express your fears with a sponsor or clergyman. Hospice usually has a chaplain available.
- ❁ Listen carefully to the dying person's wishes. Sometimes a simple change of position in the bed, the sharing of some scripture, or reading short meditations from AA literature is helpful.
- ❁ Avoid feeling "stuck." Every situation is temporary. You'll get through whatever is presented if you can focus on love, understanding and the realization that it is a privilege to help someone at this time in their life.
- ❁ If there are children in the home, be honest about the

situation, about what is happening. Talk about life and talk about death: children understand this "circle of life." Encourage them to participate in the dying person's journey, not to avoid it or run away from it. This is the time when family and friends are needed the most and they can feel important.

❂ Cry when you want to. Don't stuff your feelings. Welcome them, let them pass, and know that you are doing fine. God really doesn't give us more than we can handle in any given day. You'll feel "tested" but never abandoned. God is always there when your heart and mind are open to get you through a particular situation.

❂ Sudden death is often more difficult to handle than a slow death of cancer or another disease, which allow loved ones to have closure, to say last words to each other, to tie up "loose ends." If a friend or family member dies in an accident or by suicide, much is left unsaid, amends not made. It's important to share what you would have said to this person with a sponsor, counselor or member of the clergy.

❂ If someone dies before you can make amends, there are many ways to work Step Nine. If money is owed, give the amount to a charity. If amends need to be made, spend some time in a nursing home or with dis advantaged children in memory of that person. Visit the person's grave or write a letter. Action can lead to absolution.

❂ Remember that death is part of life. Even though it evokes sadness and grief, it also helps us feel, to be human, Being sober we feel more pain than if we could drink or drug it away, but we also experience profound joy in honoring that person by staying sober.

Health/Injury/Hospitalization

For alcoholics, health problems often mean a compromise in drugs needed for recovery, because any mood altering prescription drug can have the same effect as taking a drink.

We learn to listen to our bodies, to monitor our reactions, and to be aware of what can happen.

When Angie was newly sober, she needed some routine dental work. Her dentist had been treating her for years, so when he needed to numb an area, he gave Angie what he always did, a fast-acting type of novocaine.

"As soon as the substance hit my bloodstream, I thought, 'This must be what speed is like.' I broke out in a cold sweat, began shaking uncontrollably, and the dentist began monitoring my pulse and temperature, realizing I was having an adverse reaction to the drug. He had no idea why I was reacting differently than before."

He checked her chart and she had been given the same substance about three years prior. As he stood by her side, Angie told him about her alcoholism, how she was now sober for almost a year.

"He took my chart and wrote in red that I was never to be given anything with a fast-acting ingredient," she said. "I began to calm down and return to normal after about a half-hour of what for me was sheer terror. To this day, he allows extra time to give me plain old novocaine, which has no side effect on me. When I had to visit an oral surgeon to have a tooth removed, his office conveyed my allergies and the procedure was done with regular novocaine."

Many over-the-counter drugs have alcohol or substances that can cause a faster pulse or, conversely, make you sleepy. It's important as a recovering person to always read the label and follow directions, something none of us really gave much thought to in our active drinking days. If it feels good, double the dose!

***

When Angie was 13 years sober, she needed arthroscopic surgery on her knee. She made sure the anesthesiologist knew she was an alcoholic and requested that she be monitored carefully during the period where she obviously would have no control. When it was over and pain pills were prescribed, she requested that, instead of a huge supply, she be given enough for a few days with a refill if she needed more.

"I did not need any more than the original amount prescribed, and my request eliminated narcotics in the house as a temptation to myself or others. I knew I had the option of throwing the rest away, but that REALLY goes against the grain of an alcoholic, in recovery or not. No matter how long I am sober, the mind games still play, even if I am 'just an alcoholic' who didn't try drugs, not even pot. I have to continually remind myself that I've become a pickle, never to be a cucumber again. I have to avoid 'stinking thinking,' to be ever-vigilant of my day-at-a-time program.

***

Perhaps the most difficult situation arose three years later when she was faced with total knee replacement. In the three years since the original out-patient surgery, the cartilage had totally deteriorated and Angie had constant pain.

"I would be walking along and suddenly fall down, then would have to painfully jiggle my knee to get it into position so I could stand and walk again. When I realized I couldn't trust my knee in picking up my first grandbaby, I decided to take my orthopedic surgeon's advice and have it replaced," she said, adding that she had been advised it would never get better, only worse, and the sooner she had the operation the better.

"My mother had asked that I get a second opinion," she laughed. "I told her that I could give my OWN second opinion, looking at the x-rays of my good and bad knees. The bad, right one, didn't even look human."

This time it was not out-patient surgery. It meant preparation, donating her own blood in case it would be needed, and many other pre-op procedures.

"At each step along the way in the month prior to the surgery, I made every doctor and health care person aware of my concerns and allergy to mood-altering substances," she said. "Each person assured me I would be okay, making notes on my chart. I experienced a tremendous amount of fear prior to the surgery, asking myself many 'what if' questions. The only way to alleviate the mounting anxiety was to face the situation."

She talked at length with the anesthesiologist, because this would be a much longer, more detailed surgery.

"It was rather frightening, knowing that they would be sawing off two important leg bones to insert a metal prosthesis," she said. "I had nightmares that the new leg wouldn't be long enough."

The surgery went well, and when she came to, Angie was hooked to a morphine "drip."

"Because of my alcoholic history, I was concerned, but I never felt a high or a low from it. I was told it was taking care of the pain, that controls had been put in so I couldn't over-medicate," she said, adding that there were times when she would have taken it all at once, the pain was so great. After four days, the morphine was stopped and other medication was given, monitored carefully to take care of the pain, not to give her a reaction.

"In contrast, the woman next to me in the room, who had the same surgery, was delirious, loud and crazy after her operation, demanding more and more drugs," she said. "I was able to face all the pain with a certain degree of dignity because I was sober."

Angie was grateful for her program, for the many AAs who came to visit, and for the ability to meditate during painful moments.

"I won't say I didn't cry, scream at the therapists or wish I had never done it, but with the help of the program and the people in AA, I got through the tough few days after the surgery," she said. "And, as in the previous surgery, I requested minimum amounts of pain killers."

The best solution was the wonderful "ice machine" they sent home with her to keep the swelling down and pain at a tolerable level. Within a couple of weeks Angie was off pain killers, keeping the discomfort in control with over-the-counter meds.

"I did require a pain killer prior to each physical therapy session, however," she said. "They were excruciating!"

Angie was told that when she was on the operating table, the surgeon could not get her leg to zero degrees, that is, totally straight. She had been favoring the leg for so long her hamstring and sciatic nerve had actually shrunk.

"The therapists were concerned that I would never be able to totally straighten the leg," she said. "That's all this alcoholic had to hear. If I went through all this misery, pain and grief, I was damn well going to have "zero degrees."

It took six months of gruelling therapy, but Angie did

it. The only problem she still has is that the leg doesn't bend as far as she would like, making it impossible to safely ride a regular bike through the neighborhood. Other than that, she's pretty well back to "normal" in terms of the leg.

"Now I can obsess on the NEXT time it has to be done, because it only lasts for so many years," she said. "I'll have to go through the whole procedure again. I try not to project, to worry about the future, but being an alcoholic, I sometimes have problems staying in the day. It's then that I ask God to take all these silly thoughts away and help me concentrate on what I'm supposed to do this moment in this day. After all, I might be dead before I have to get another knee. In the meantime, I'll live it up."

Angie saw the surgery on television a few years after the knee was replaced.

"If I had seen it prior to having the operation, I don't know that I could have given the go-ahead for the surgery," she said. "You are never told how difficult or painful it really is."

Recently the osteoarthritis necessitated arthroscopic surgery on Angie's left knee, which she jokes is about "10 years behind the right knee." With the advance in technology, she only needed one pain pill after surgery and was off crutches almost immediately with no significant pain.

Gaining on Pain – A Delicate Balance

Connie has had to learn to live with constant pain. She doesn't know if some is the result of her early drinking and taking pills, or if it's her genetic make-up coupled with age. She has a litany of problems: diabetes, peripheral neuropathy, high blood pressure, depression, and she's had three mini strokes. Trying to keep her sanity as well as her sobriety under the necessity of taking several different drugs has complicated her life. Many times, she has called Angie to tell her what she has taken and asked her to call back in a bit to make sure she is okay. The pain is constant, with some days easier than others. She does what she can. She has the fear of "getting hooked" and not wanting to take her meds. She has often delayed taking certain drugs because of her conditioning in AA that you don't take narcotic drugs. She tells doctors when she has a reaction.

"After all my years of sobriety and the things I've dealt with, one thing is sure: I don't want to get drunk again, on booze or pills," she said.

Connie has looked at alternative ways to deal with the pain, but in her words, "they don't work." It's a real program tester. But then, so is life. She heard them say early in sobriety that we were not being promised a rose garden, but that we were being presented a workable set of tools. For the first time in her life, she felt herself growing into a responsible adult.

Before AA Connie was going around in circles and didn't know it. Now when she starts "going around in circles" she knows it's because she's an alcoholic who chooses not to take a drink or drug today to alter her mind. Meditation, prayer, people in the program – these are her true drugs of choice today. They are the ones that work.

"Part of my daily prayer when I came into AA was for God to give me one second of sanity between the thought and the action.," she said. "That's where I am today, despite having to take medications."

Before, she never paid attention to herself. Today she's the most important person in her life with a strong, workable program to take care of herself.

When Nothing Seems to Work

Several of Angie's recovering women friends suffer from fibromyalgia, a debilitating condition that delivers extreme pain to the connective tissues or muscles.

"I never really feel good," said Carol. "It's like having the flu all the time, similar to having chronic fatigue syndrome except that you hurt all the time."

Very little is known about the disease, so Carol uses the program to survive.

What she does in a day correlates to how much pain she is in.

"If I'm moving around fairly easy with a pain level of four, I plan to do more things because I know I'll be able to," she explained. "If it's a pain level of six, I know I have to be efficient because I'll run out of fuel."

While medication has been prescribed, Carol didn't notice much difference in the intensity of her pain, but felt dulled, slowed down.

"I've found that using God to help remove the pain is more powerful than any medication I've been given," she said. "I ask for the strength to walk through it. Sometimes my thinking is affected by the pain, and that's as much of a fog as I want to experience. I want to be as fresh and alert as possible. Taking drugs isn't worth what I lose in my cognitive ability."

She values quiet time and has simplified her life. She has a beautiful lavender bedroom and her home overlooks a small lake with terraces to the water. She enjoys meditating, filling herself with serenity and keeping a positive attitude day to day.

"I store my energy like a battery," she said. "When I have it to use I do. When I need recharging I take care of myself to allow my strength to return. I've learned to live with the pain and concentrate on everything that's positive in my life. It's not easy, but that's how I've stayed sober for many years. I've found that God is the best prescription possible and the only one that works."

Still a 'Pickle'

After almost 23 years of continuous sobriety Angie still occasionally has the feeling of being in a black hole, of not caring about anyone, thinking that it would be better to just end everything.

"It bothers me that these negative thoughts can overrun any sensible way of looking at reality," she said, shaking her head. "Even when I know in my mind that things will eventually work out, I am overpowered by the emotional dread and fear that they won't. I get so tired, so overwhelmed, particularly with financial matters, that I can hardly cope. Yet it only takes a spark of positive news to bring me around again to acceptance and trust that God is truly taking care of me."

She said she doesn't think about drinking, but sometimes has thoughts of suicide as the "easier, softer way" when she's feeling down.

"I let the thought consciously pass through my head, knowing I will not act," she said. "Sometimes it amuses me that an old pattern can rear up to produce a knee jerk reaction to what is happening in my life at the moment. It's usually something insignificant in the great scheme of things that challenges my security or self esteem: someone has spoken to me in a harsh tone of voice, my children didn't do as I expected or ignored my good advice, I was overcharged on a bill, or something didn't happen as promised. I am not even aware that I sometimes mentally set myself up for a negative reaction."

It is then that she once again is made aware of alcoholism as a form of mental illness.

"The thought of suicide isn't normal thinking," she said. "Verbalizing to my sponsor and writing about my feelings always helps a negative cycle pass. Being aware of my patterns and how I spontaneously deal with various situations help me put them into perspective. Nothing is that upsetting or important today to risk my sobriety. I thank God that I know what's wrong with me and I thank Him for giving me solutions. It's that simple."

I can't, He can, I think I'll let Him.

Suggestions for handling health problems

- ❂ Be sure that all health care providers, your doctor, your dentist, know you are alcoholic. Do this verbally, not in writing on any form that may hurt your insurance coverage. If you're sober, you're not drinking and alcohol is not a current problem What's past is past.
- ❂ Read labels on over-the-counter drugs and other products. Even mouth washes and cough syrups contain alcohol.
- ❂ Read labels for warnings and follow the directions. This is hard if we're alcoholic because we don't want to be told what to do and not do, even on a label!
- ❂ If you are given a prescription drug that triggers your addiction, call your doctor immediately. There is usually a non-addictive alternative that can be prescribed.
- ❂ Be aware of your body. Years of drinking have taught us to abuse ourselves, to think nothing of hurting ourselves. Today we can take care of and value our health – physically, emotionally and mentally.
- ❂ If we are having unusual stress or recurring pain as a result of stress consider all the options, including counseling, massage, relaxation therapy, listening to soothing music and, most important, prayer.
- ❂ If you have a chronic illness, ask God to help with

your condition, to relieve pain and to help you keep a positive attitude. Drinking will never make a condition better, only worse.

❀ Always be aware that alcoholism is a form of mental illness that can produce an unhealthy mood and negative thoughts. Get positive again through meditation, talking with a sponsor or going to a meeting. The longer you're "down" the more difficult it will be to get "up."

Relationships

I wonder...Is the need for daily contact with a man similar to maintenance drinking? The need for a fix, a "feel good" input...is the emotional need similar to physical need? A relationship is like another substance if we are not well. The thought "If he would just call" can be translated "If I could just have one drink." The call could trigger the need for more, it would never be enough. The thought that "next time it will be different" is futile. It leads to a downward spiral to an emotional bottom of acute loneliness looking for a "fix."
Angie's writings 1987

Of all subjects, relationships probably get more alcoholics in trouble than anything else mentioned. Because relationships touch our interaction with every other human being, from small child to business person, to friend or romantic partner, it is all encompassing. Relationships touch the core of our emotions. How other people react to us, interpret our words or actions, view us physically, respond to our body language or visible feelings – all play a role in whether or not we stay sober.

Sponsees often rebel when sponsors advise, "No romantic relationship in the first year." It is particularly dangerous if they are at the "pink cloud" state of mind where they think everything in life is okay now because they've stopped drinking. Certainly the right partner would make life complete. Wrong. Only steadfast sobriety, working the steps and following all the suggestions doled out by a sponsor and in the AA literature will make life "complete."

Angie reminded a sponsee who was desperately hoping a relationship would work that someone can't give what isn't there.

"If someone, man or woman, cannot love themselves and be comfortable in their own skin, there is no way they can love someone else in an emotionally mature relationship," she said. "It just isn't going to happen."

So, when alcoholic woman meets alcoholic man (we tend to repeat patterns...hopefully this time both are sober!) they are on a collision course that spans every conceivable emotion. The relationship not only involves the obvious physical merry-go-round of boy-meets-girl, there is all the other "stuff" thrown in from the past: ex-'s, children, finances, differing goals, opinions, sponsors, and, of course, hormones which can disrupt any aspect of involvement with someone of the opposite sex. There are tremendous changes going on, particularly for the woman.

She may be on her own for the first time. She may be drowning in loneliness and abandonment without even realizing it. A "rescuer" would be very tempting. Because our social contact is usually limited to work and AA meetings the first year, the knight in shining armor may be sitting in the rooms in his own sea of loneliness (although he probably won't be able to clearly recognize or admit his own emotional state) just waiting for the chance to "save" a vulnerable woman. It is doubtful that either party is, at this point, asking what God's will is for them.

You bring me roses.
Are you just another face for my fantasy
Or is this one wrapped in reality?
It's so hard to tell
When loneliness shadows needs and wants.
Angie's writings 1986

Nancy admitted she married the first man in the program who kissed her on the neck one night and who gave her a spectacular orgasm soon after – something she had never experienced in 22 years of addiction while with her ex-husband.

We don't always think with our head in times like this. If it feels good, many women in early sobriety will go for it, "thinking" (rationalizing) this must be the next "right" thing to do.

Angie pointed out that before women get sober our emotions have been diluted or drowned with alcohol.

"We were basically numb.," said Angie. "Feelings were dulled or evident only when we were drunk and uninhibited, if we can remember them at all. Some women never had sex without a drink. How in the world can they handle a 'first time' experience after sobriety? The very thought can scare the beejeebees out of us!"

Once we have a foothold on sobriety after the first year or so, the best suggestion is to take it easy, despite the tendency to rush in when we think we've found the right person. If he IS right, then taking some time to make sure (and praying together) will make it all the better. Respect has to come before love, first by respecting ourselves, then by earning it from another person.

"Setting boundaries and avoiding expectations nurtures self respect," said Angie. "It becomes important what WE do, not what someone else does."

He says he'll call
I arrange and change
And another day goes by.
"What are you going to do? he asks.
"Nothing," I say.
"If both people do nothing, how does anything begin?"

There's a twinkle in his eye.

I slip into denial once again. That old feeling of am I worth it and do I deserve this and what does he really think of me and will that twinkle still be there when a mood swing slaps me from behind and I am again faced with who and what I am and what I have? Will he be able to hold me and tell me it's okay and love me because of who and what I am? Will I be there in turn when he has a bad day? If we're both stuck at once will we have the courage to turn to God instead of each other until it passes and the twinkle in his eye returns?

Angie's writings 1987

When a woman reaches the point where she needs someone because she WANTS him instead of wanting him because she NEEDS him, then maybe it's safe to proceed, to let God unfold a new level of happiness.

Angie cautions sponsees who have gone through the 12 Steps to "practice these principles in all their affairs." If the steps are applied to a relationship between recovering alcoholics, it has a good chance of surviving and thriving.

But what about the woman who gets sober and manages to stay married to a loving, caring partner who may not be alcoholic? This is a perfect situation for that partner to attend Al-Anon meetings to get the support he'll need to also grow in this new relationship, because no matter if they've been married for 20 years, it is a new situation. The marriage will be enriched by both growing spiritually, which will in turn have a wonderful effect on every family member. Sobriety gives everyone another chance.

***

Angie pointed out that it was important for her to take time for herself after her divorce, to attend to her children, her business and life in general.

"I wasn't opposed to someone coming into my life, but I also wasn't looking. I figured if it happened it happened."

As shared earlier in this book, she met a man in the program two years after her divorce who died within 14 months of cancer, a journey that left a lasting impression.

"I was grateful to have the chance to love on this level, and truthfully felt no one else would be able to fill that void again," she said. "While I kept an eye out for someone interesting, it never happened. I had a few dates here and there, but I learned later from an older man friend in AA that I terrified most program men because I had my own business, paid my own bills, was not needy and gave the illusion that I really didn't WANT anyone in my life. I told him I really DID want someone, but that I wasn't willing to settle. Living in a large city made no difference. I might as well have been living in cow town USA for all the emotionally available men I met. They were either taken or gay."

As her children left the nest she realized she didn't want to be alone. But she also didn't want to have to go through all the hoops to "find" someone. She would often say, jokingly, "I don't want to date, I just want to find someone and marry him." The chase, the hunt, the "game" really didn't interest her at this stage in life. She didn't want to waste time and wanted to avoid the emotional trauma/hassle that a new relationship always creates.

"When I was sober 17 years after 17 years of drinking, I felt I might be ready to find a mate, a companion, a lover, a buddy for the rest of my life," she said. "But how was I to find someone when I worked at home, most of my business partners and contacts were also involved with my son, and my social life evolved around AA meetings?"

She said she literally "lives" on the computer. All her work is done on it, she's on constant email and it is her connection to the outside world.

So she turned to high tech.

"I had placed some personal ads over the years just as a joke to see who would respond, met a few men for lunch and decided I had to get a little more specific on who/what I was looking for," she said. "I created a screen name that I used only for this purpose that could not be traced to me personally. Then I took a leap. I realized I was putting in an order for someone, so this is the ad I placed (without a photo):

So tired of all the BS normally dished out. I'm a young 53, successful, sober professional with my own business and lots going for myself. Would like to meet a kind, compassionate, successful guy, preferably someone who's into flying, sailing, water sports. I'm 5'7" so would prefer someone 5'11" or taller, but am more concerned with what's "inside" than outside appearances. I like traveling, spending time in the Bahamas, have two grown kids, one grandchild and a dog. I've got tons of interests. If you are not married and have been on your own awhile, are sober, don't smoke or do drugs and can be totally honest, please respond. I don't expect a big rush of replies!

She then said, "Okay, God...YOU find him," and pretty much treated the ad as a game. She had a few responses from men who obviously couldn't read, which she graciously (!) pointed out since they couldn't identify her, and amused herself with how desperate, macho and stupid some men can be.

Then one day she got the response, "Check out my profile. If interested, please respond."

"He was six years older than me, divorced, unattached, stated he was interested in sailing, flying, classical guitar, photography and writing, that he was a retired high school English teacher who now worked for local government. He lived about an hour away. His favorite selected personal quote: 'This above all – to thine own self be true...thou canst not then be false to any man.'"

She recognized the quote from what was engraved on many of the time marker medallions she had received in AA meetings over the years.

Mmm. He hadn't mentioned music or photography, but both were important in Angie's life. She had majored in English and creative writing. She was also pleased that he had a Macintosh computer instead of a PC.

"When you're searching for that needle, it helps to have a bigger magnifying glass, so I said, 'Okay, God, let's go,' and answered him.

Over the next few weeks of "You've got mail!" Angie and her new friend got to know each other.

"While we discovered we have a lot in common, including sobriety – he with six years at the time, we also are very different, an attraction of opposites. I am a risk taker and tend to be spontaneous. In one of his emails he said he was spontaneous 'once in 1987.' While I worked for employers for only short times in my career, he, while wanting to have his own business, required the security of such things as dental insurance."

They discussed their children (he has a daughter and a granddaughter) and past relationships. Angie was pleased when he admitted he was not a "fool-around" kind of guy, that he had been in a 25-year marriage and a 10-year relationship in the past.

Because they hadn't yet met in person, the relationship was purely objective. While emotions evolved during "mail" conversations back and forth almost every night, she said nothing could be "acted" on.

"It was a safe environment to get to know someone indirectly (we didn't even tell each other our names for a week)," she said. "We were able to more easily explore our feelings, likes and dislikes, ideas, hopes and fears. We learned that we were of different political persuasions, which to this day makes for some tippy-toeing away from certain issues."

They shared every aspect of their lives, their dreams, disappointments, failures and successes.

"We discussed petty peeves with the people around us, and became comfortable as good friends," she said. "After about three weeks we exchanged photos so we could envision the person on the other computer."

Then came the day they were to meet in person.

"THAT was a biggy," she laughed. "Here we were, two people who had gotten to know each other electronically on an intellectual level without a clue how we would react to each other in person."

Wanting as safe a situation as possible, they decided on a movie, dinner and an AA meeting for their first date.

"He admits he was afraid to get off the exit to my house, and I admit I was scared to open the door. My dog, the type that many fear as a guard dog, was also anxious, sensing my uneasiness," she said. "As he came into the room, my dog perched on the back of the sofa which extends into the room, gently took his right arm in her mouth, and walked him along the couch into the room, as if to warn, 'Don't try anything, Buster!' It was a great icebreaker, giving us both a laugh. Then my dog seemed to sense everything was okay, that she no longer had to protect me."

He had passed the first "test."

There were, of course, many more tests as they got to know each other and eventually put all their "stuff" in Angie's house and became a couple.

"Because he did not fit my past pattern of men and I am not like his previous emotionally destructive dysfunctional partners, the relationship has worked a day at a time for a few years now," she said. "In the beginning we had to hire a dog psychologist to bring his two dogs and a cat into an environment where my dog ruled, but even that has worked out. The cat enjoys her own room in the house, safely viewing the dog through French door windows."

With both of them in the program at different stages of sobriety, it hasn't been easy juggling emotions, intentions, sensitivity and goals.

"Our differences are enormous at times, but we are no longer afraid to confront them. If something isn't clear, we ask what the other means rather than guessing."

Angie said she has a habit of scrunching up her face when he says something that doesn't make sense to her at the moment, which he finds offensive.

"He often looks mad at the world, with a disturbing crease in his forehead," she said. "I know today it has nothing to do with me, but in the beginning we had to talk about how we react to inner emotions portrayed on the outside, whether in facial expressions or body language. In the past I would ignore the signals. Today I am not afraid to find out the meaning behind them and to risk approval or disapproval from my mate."

She said the important thing is knowing that neither of them is perfect and that their intentions are never to hurt one another.

"This has led to understanding, tolerance, patience, forgiveness and love for one another," she said. "Communication is the key. When both people in a relationship are on the same page differences disappear."

Suggestions for relationships

❀ Try to stay focused on recovery in the first year, avoiding emotional involvement with someone new. If you are married or in a relationship with a significant other, communicate that you need extra time for yourself, for meetings, and a sponsor. Encourage them to explore Al-Anon.

❀ It's important to learn to live by yourself and be responsible for yourself/children before entering into a new relationship. By getting healthy you will have a good chance of a healthy future relationship because you will not "settle" for the same old situation.

❀ When you think you are ready for a relationship but still have some fear or doubts, use the internet anonymously to see if someone in cyberspace fits what you're looking for. Be specific and most of all, have fun. If you don't have expectations, you won't be disappointed. This is a good way to build self esteem and establish boundaries. A word of caution: GO SLOW!

❀ When God wants us to find someone it will happen if we're not needy or desperate. Take your time, be aware, and know that you are worthy of love and a caring partner.

❀ Make a list of all the characteristics you would like in a mate, concentrating on how you want him to be

rather than how you want him to look. Kindness, consideration and compassion are far more important than looks.
✿ Be up front about being sober. No surprises, no disappointments later. Be proud of your sobriety – value it as your most precious asset.

Career/Finances

When we get sober, we come from a variety of work and career backgrounds. For some of us, recovery means changing how we earn a living, particularly if we worked in the entertainment or hospitality markets as bar maids, waitresses, bartenders or in the gaming industry, where liquor and money flow constantly.

We may be professionals or homemakers. Alcohol has no favorites, its victims come from all walks, ages and stages of life. If stress is a normal part of the job, we may find that we need to find work that gives us more serenity. Perhaps we always wanted to be _____ when we grew up. Well, now may be that time. After all, we are only as old emotionally as the day we started drinking. Many women have gone back to school, changed professions and taken leaps that would have been impossible while drinking. We are given the chance to become the person we always wanted to be, and that includes what we do to earn a living.

We are also told to avoid making major life changes in the first year of sobriety...divorce, career, relationship. If we work where alcohol is served, however, change may be necessary the day we get sober. It's called "going to any lengths" to put sobriety before everything else. Without sobriety, there may not BE a job.

Angie feels she is fortunate to have begun her own business "before they burned the bra" and that she was able to continue in the same business when she got sober.

"I was able to do a better job and give clients the time they deserved," she said. "In my drinking days, I often had to reschedule appointments because I was hung over, robbing them of their time and causing them to alter their schedules. Once sober, I could manage appointments, be more creative, get referrals for new clients, and do a much better job than before."

But there came a time when, through no fault of Angie's, that she was forced to change her business.

"I could no longer place news releases with my primary source for income, and overnight I had to change from public relations writing to advertising and design in order to make a living and support my children," she said, a fearful expression on her face. "This happened eight years into sobriety. I can't imagine how it would have been had I been forced to change my entire business right after treatment, so I can empathize with women who have to seek different careers or jobs to survive as sober women."

Having her own business also results in a lot of "down" days that don't always get balanced by "up" days.

"Learning to apply one-day-at-a-time principles to my business helps me when it's teetering back and forth," she said. "I also know that having my own business means accepting the risks that go with being an entrepreneur."

All You Have to do is Dream...

Jan got sober in her thirties. When she was 18 she had started college, but living at home was too painful. She had been sexually abused by her father from the time she was five until she was 15 years old. It was time to escape. She went to California and after a couple of geographical moves ended up in Florida. A marriage ended in divorce, leaving her a single mother struggling to survive. Her dream of college may as well have been in another lifetime.

She worked during the day in an office and as a bar maid at night while raising a son. When he was eight years old he told her he was sorry she was always so sad. It worried her that he was aware of her drinking, but she couldn't stop. A younger sister was also aware of her drinking and inquired about where AA meetings were held. She took Jan to her first two AA meetings, not knowing too much about the program, then told her she was on her own. After a couple of tries, Jan decided she would at least try this new, sober way of living.

She soon found herself able to survive financially with her day job. Eventually she married a recovering alcoholic and her son graduated high school. Life was really satisfying, but Jan found herself still haunted by her dream of going to college. When she was several years sober and working full time, she began pursuing her dream. She enrolled in a university and, a few years later, accomplished her goal. In her mid-fifties, she graduated with a four-year degree – not necessarily to use it in her career, but to fulfill a life-long dream.

"I could never have done this without getting sober first," she said. "It gave me immeasurable self-esteem and self-worth."

She encourages any woman in recovery to pursue her dream. It IS possible to accomplish what may seem to be an impossible goal – as long as sobriety comes first.

A Wrong Way and a Right Way

Anne got sober at the early age of 20 and admits she did "everything wrong." At nine months sober she switched sponsors, home group and got engaged. A week after her first anniversary she married a newly sober alcoholic and within a short time moved from the comfort of her Midwestern meetings to a U.S. military base in Germany.

"Instead of seven to 15 meetings a week, there were only three, with no women," she said. "We stayed sober by helping other couples looking for help, doing 12-step work just like the Big Book suggests, but it wasn't easy. I missed my old meetings."

After their return to the U.S., she realized how incompatible they were. He was content to sit home and read, while she had a zest for life. After five years, they amicably divorced, with the blessings of his mother.

"She was 16 years sober and played an intricate role in my sobriety," she said. "She told me I didn't have to be in a marriage where I was unhappy. She shared her experience and strength with me, and basically gave me permission to divorce her son."

Anne pursued her profession of teaching gymnastics to children, but knew she wanted to do something more with her life.

"I was offered the position of director of gymnastics where I worked. I had topped out in my field as a gymnastics teacher, and realized the position would be more responsibility than I could handle if I were to make any major life changes. " she said. "My choices were to either have my own school or get INTO school. Everything inside told me to get educated, so I worked to pay off my credit cards to simplify my life, then enrolled as a full-time student while staying a full-time gymnastics teacher."

The miracles soon began to unfold. She got a scholarship she didn't apply for, was able to get student loans, and her employer was willing to work with her school hours. Financially she could fulfill her dreams.

With a love for math and science, Anne is majoring in civil and environmental engineering with a minor in physics. She has no idea where this path will ultimately lead, but her goal is to do what she loves.

"The program has taught me to do what I'm supposed to do without worrying about the outcome. Education is the key to success, especially for women. I hope to further my income with more opportunities. Education will open doors. If my motives are right, it will all come together."

She envisions a career in quantum physics research, which she says is a "quantum leap." When asked what quantum physics is all about, she gave an example of a study done on monkeys on different islands who learned to do different things at the same time with no physical connection between the groups. Not something to comprehend without sobriety!

"When I was drinking, clothes, sex and booze gave me what I needed," she said. "My values and goals have changed. I know if I want something in life, I have to do the legwork. I also know it will provide emotional balance and self-esteem as I succeed."

After being on her own for a couple of years, she met someone in the program who is also pursuing his dreams. They've looked at rings and Anne is happy.

"We both want children and with love and a lot of faith, our lives will unfold as we both finish our degrees and begin life together."

She said this time she's "doing everything right."

Suggestions for career and financial situations

- ❁ Put sobriety first. If you have a job that would jeopardize staying sober, such as in the entertainment field, look for a change. God will help you if you ask for help.
- ❁ Go back over your life and think about all the things you wanted to do when you grew up. If alcohol robbed you of those dreams, find a way to fulfill them, no matter what age you are now.
- ❁ Learn how to budget, to control what you spend based on what you make, because financial anxiety can stress staying sober. Many women sometimes don't have a clue on where the money goes because someone else has taken care of them. In sobriety we can have a clear head and look at our situation realistically.
- ❁ Start saving, building a nest egg for the future. Setting aside the amount of only one drink a day can add up.
- ❁ No matter how tired we are at the end of a long working day, it's important to go to meetings. Remember that without sobriety there probably wouldn't be a good job. Staying active in the program preserves your new way of life. We drank no matter what. Now we have to stay sober no matter what.

"God" Stories

At some point in recovery, we become aware of a Higher Power, a God of our understanding, being present in our daily lives.

In Step Three, we decide to turn our will and our lives over to His care. Our initial reaction may well be, "What an order! I can't go through with it."

Turning it over, letting go, Thy will not mine...however we want to approach getting out of our own way, it must be done at some point for successful recovery. Angie's favorite approach is still "I can't, He can, I think I'll let Him."

But until we actually experience an "awakening" or a "message" or see God working in other people's lives, we are often skeptical that it is a truth of the program. We are encouraged by our sponsors and at meetings to be honest, open and willing for God to work in our lives. Believing will eventually lead to experiencing. This may or may not happen in early recovery, but when we are faced with a crisis, a crucial life decision or a total sense of helplessness in a given situation, the answer will be there if we ask for God's help.

Angie mentioned again how she had been raised Catholic and had chucked "religion" per se at the end of her drinking. In recovery, she developed a new "God," a friend who could be called on when she desperately needed an answer to something she just couldn't handle on her own. While sitting in meetings, she has heard many "God" stories from women. Personally, she had three specific incidents she wanted to share.

"When I was sober about five years, a situation arose where I had to find a special school for my son to deal with a specific learning disability. I had done everything I could for him at that point, and I knew it was necessary to let go of him, to find a boarding school," she said. "But I was not in the financial position to provide what he needed. When we found a school that was right for him, the cost was prohibitive. I agonized over how I would meet this child's special needs. One day I got on my knees, put my head in my hands on my bed, and sobbed, asking for God to please help me with the solution to this seemingly overwhelming problem. I stayed still for some time until the tears subsided and I felt calm. My father had been dead for almost six years, but I felt his presence, and I heard him say 'the trust.'"

Angie's parents had always been very private people when it came to money or inheritance. She said none of the six children were ever told about her father's final decision on inheritance prior to or after his death.

"I did know, however, that trust funds had been set up for grandchildren for college," she said. "That's all I was told, not how much or any other detail. I also knew that it was quite possible my son would never be able to use his trust because it was highly improbable that he would GO to college. My only request of him was that he graduate high school. At the time, there was no help in the public or private local schools for a dyslexic. If he was going to get a high school diploma, we had to find another way."

For months she had been sharing the situation with her mother, who went with Angie and her son on a couple of interviews at out-of-state schools.

"When I took my son to the school he ultimately attended, I sensed the same relief in him that a newcomer feels when discovering AA," she said. "Finally there's help!"

She called her mother after getting the "message" from her father and her mother shared that at the very same time, she felt compelled to look over the trust papers for the grandchildren.

"My mother said it wasn't just for college, that the money could be used for the child's 'needs,' and that she certainly recognized the need at hand. It was a miracle and the help we needed."

Her son attended the school for two-and-a-half years, long enough to get the foundation he needed to ultimately graduate high school. He joined the U.S. Navy, spent 18 months in the Persian Gulf during the crisis, and one day called Angie collect from some distant Asian port.

"He asked if I was sitting down. I told him that it was in the middle of the night and that I was in bed. He said he had something important to tell me. I sat up, wondering what had happened now. He told me he had just scored the highest on a test for material one level above what he had actually studied for."

This did not surprise her because, even though handicapped with dyslexia, she knew her son was brilliant.

"If he took an oral test, he always scored high. But this time, he told me he had taken a 'bubble' test, the type where you read something on one sheet and fill in the circle on an answer sheet, an almost impossible task for a classic dyslexic. He told me that something miraculous must have taken place, that he had 'jumped' the short circuit in his brain which now seemed to function normally."

Her son went on to take a college entrance exam (another "bubble" variety) and was one in 25 accepted to begin college aboard the Navy ship.

"Although he didn't continue college, he proved he could do it," she said, smiling. "Today he owns a successful graphics and printing business. Occasionally he'll make an error and wink, 'What do you expect from a dyslexic?' Talk about gratitude – sometimes I am overwhelmed."

Another situation arose when she was about nine years sober. She has a little house in the Bahamas which she began renting out after buying her ex-'s half.

"The slow season is the fall, and in the early days of raising the children and making ends meet, I questioned if I was doing the right thing holding on to this wonderful little place," she said. "As my financial situation worsened, I did the only thing I knew to do. I got on my knees as I had done in the crisis with my son and asked God to please help me, to give me a sign, to tell me if I was holding on to this property for selfish reasons or if it was what He wanted me to do."

Again, she experienced a sense of calm after crying out, and totally dismissed the problem from her mind. She truly "turned it over."

About two weeks later, Angie received a phone call on a Sunday afternoon from a previous renter.

"I know it was Sunday because he always called during business hours and I remember being surprised by the call and the tone of his voice," she said. "He apologized for the weekend interruption and explained that he was compelled to call to ask me a question. I encouraged him to continue."

He began talking about how he had read a "Blue Book" at her island house two years ago when it had rained for the few days he was there. After a long silence Angie began to shake. He asked if she was in the program.

"I told him yes, that I was several years sober now, and that the name of my house reflected all the promises of the program."

He told her that the next year he rented, it also rained and that he had read the "Blue Book" again. After a long silence, he quietly shared that as a result, he had gotten sober two months ago and just wanted her to know.

"The hair stood on my arm, we both started crying, and I had my answer," she said. "I was to keep the house, that financially I would survive, and that it was to be there, in the middle of nowhere, as a refuge to alcoholics."

Since that time she has answered many VHF radio calls from cruising yachties looking for a "friend of Bill W." Meetings often include a friend in recovery who lives on the island, a loner listed in the international directory of AA. Angie's "Blue Book" and 12-and-12 are on the bookshelf with a motley collection of paperbacks left by former renters. They are there for anyone who needs them.

The Signs Were Everywhere!

Maryanne has some wonderful God stories. She always believed in God, but didn't think He would have anything to do with her because she had so much shame, remorse and guilt. She prayed, but didn't expect any answers because she felt so unworthy.

When she was newly sober and out of treatment in November 1989, her daughter asked what she wanted for Christmas. Maryanne told her "something with the praying hands on it." She looked everywhere and couldn't find anything, so Maryanne also went on the mission, searching stores for a pin, necklace, anything with the praying hands. In tears, she decided that if God wanted her to have it He'd provide. When she arrived home, there was a Christmas card on the table from someone she hadn't wanted to talk to. The praying hands were attached to the card. She screamed, "Thank you, God!" She laughs today that sometimes a two-year-old mentality can be a blessing.

Another time in early sobriety she was driving down a busy street crying, depressed over her situation. A car went past that had a "One Day At a Time" bumper sticker. It got her attention. The very next car that passed said "Easy Does It," then another went by that said "Let Go and Let God." She looked up and said, "God, is that You?" Then to test Him, she said, "You know I'm an alcoholic and addict Lord, can I just have one more?" At that point a stinking garbage truck pulled in front of her with a big hand that said "Just Say No To Drugs." She was going to turn at the intersection, feeling much better and cracking up over all her "signs." But God had the last word. The car coming toward her had a front license plate that said "Smile, God loves you." Insignificant? We don't think so.

Another time people from her AA group invited her to a church. She was listening to the pastor when he stopped in the middle of a prayer and said, "My child, I brought you here today because I love you. I don't care where you've been or what you've done, just give me your disease and come home." It touched her so deeply that she began crying. "It was like the dam broke," she said. "I don't know how long I stood there crying before I realized I was the only person standing. I remember that it didn't matter that everyone looked at me, or what they thought about me." It was insignificant at the time.

She recalls thinking that in the presence of God there is no ego. "It was the most wonderful awakening, to learn that day that ego is where all the pain comes from," she said. Maryanne saw it as a reconciliation with the God she thought would have nothing to do with her. She was no longer separated, she was connected to God. She recalls that being spiritually separated was so horrible, that she felt so alone, she never wants to be separated from God again.

Ask, And You Shall Receive

When Judy went to her first AA meeting, she was so "pumped up" she wanted to go on a diet, quit smoking and write everyone she knew. She was told to concentrate on her sobriety the first year and that everything else would happen in due time if it was in God's plan. After drinking, she was primarily concerned about smoking, because she began drinking and smoking at the same time.

As she worked on her sobriety through the steps, she asked God if he would help her with the smoking after a year. Her anniversary came and went. Then one Saturday she was quite sick with a headache. She could barely move.

"Instead of the almost two packs of cigarettes a day I was smoking, I only had one or two," she said. The next day she had a cigarette, and as she lit up the second one, she heard a very strong voice say, "Today is the day you're going to stop smoking." It was very clear.

She said, "okay," and put it out and quit. Four years later during Hurricane Andrew, some heavy smokers were visiting.

"I was so exhausted I had a cigarette with them. There I was again, up to my usual one to two packs a day."

Her daughter, who knew she had quit four years earlier, was living with her, so Judy didn't smoke in the house. When she got "caught," her daughter pleaded with her to stop. Judy promised she would stop in 1994, two years down the line.

"At the beginning of 1994 she reminded me of my promise," she said, "but I hadn't told her WHEN in 1994."

On March 19, 1994, in the middle of smoking a cigarette, she again heard the deep voice say, "Today is the day you're going to stop smoking."

She said "okay" and put it out. That was her last cigarette.

"Both times, in August 1988 and again in March 1994, when I stopped smoking I had no withdrawals – none," she said. "I was amazed, because every time I tried to quit before getting sober I suffered from horrible withdrawals. I know that God helped me with my addiction to nicotine."

A Wheel of Fortune

My friend Connie also has many "God" stories, with one in particular standing out. She had been estranged from her sons for a few years, feeling the pain of the separation and another level of "letting go."

One morning she was feeling particularly glum. She acknowledged she had a belief in God, but wanted to *really* believe. She knew in her head that if her sons were supposed to be in her life they would be, particularly since her amends had been made, but all she got was a cold shoulder.

She got on her knees and prayed: "God, you know that I believe in you, but I'm feeling so lonely and unhappy and missing my sons. You know, God, what would help would be a little assurance. Perhaps there's a way You can show me that You are active in my life and that everything is okay."

At the end of the prayer, she got up, finished getting ready for work and left the house. As she went to her car she saw a young man walking toward her on the street. She smiled and he smiled back. They arrived at her car about the same time.

He looked down and said, "Looks like you have a flat tire, lady." She had never changed a tire in her life so was a little upset. He asked, "Would you like me to change it?"

She said, "I'd really appreciate that." He explained that he would need a ride to work so he wouldn't be late and Connie assured him, "No problem. Good deal."

He went about changing the tire and they didn't have any conversation, but between her house and his work, they started to chat. Connie again told him thank you, and said, "By the way, my name is Connie. What is yours?"

He said "Steve."

She asked his last name and he said, "Jones." She was

startled.

"That's my son's name," she said.

He told her the reason he stopped to help her was that she reminded him so much of his mother. All Connie could do was smile and say, "Thank you, God."

She never saw that young man before that day nor since.

"He just appeared out of the blue. To me, he was an angel."

***

By the time we get to Step 12, those in recovery are conscious that God often does for us what we cannot do for ourselves. The key is to let Him help us. If we hold on to a problem, it stays with us. Only by totally letting go and leaving the outcome to our Higher Power is it able to be solved.

I can't, He can, I think I'll let Him.

Suggestions for recognizing God

- When attending AA meetings, listen carefully to how God, or the Higher Power, has actually worked in the lives of others.
- When you have a problem or need an answer, kneel down, ask God to take the problem from you, to give you an answer. Then forget it, no matter how difficult this may seem.
- If you can't mentally give the problem to God, write the situation down along with the request that HE solve it. Put it in a "God jar," tighten the lid, and forget it. If your mind still races with the problem, go to your God jar, read what you wrote, put it back and start all over. Eventually, you'll not have to "take it back."
- When you think a situation is a coincidence, reflect that it might be God remaining anonymous. Smile and enjoy the process.
- Believe just because others believe that God is working in your life.

Getting Professional Help

Sometimes it becomes necessary to seek professional help beyond what we learn in 12 Step programs. We may be able to stop drinking by getting a sponsor and going to meetings, but a sponsor is not a professional. Sponsors can only share their experiences, strength and hope of their own recovery. If, after doing the steps, there is still discomfort, guilt, doubt or deep-seated issues such as co-dependence, sexual and/or emotional abuse or severe family dysfunction, it may be necessary to work with a professional to free ourselves of those debilitating problems. At this point it is normal to feel extremely sensitive and vulnerable, which makes it crucial to choose the right professional, as the following story illustrates.

Rebecca's story is a journey that could have totally destroyed her – her sobriety, her career, her emotional well-being, possibly her very life. It was through the strength of her program, women in AA and a conviction to "do the right thing" that she was able to tell her story. It spans a five year period that began with abuse by a clergyman and led to realization, accusation, prosecution and finally, resolution. Looking back, she knows God gave her the strength to do what she could not do by herself. It's a story that is all too common yet hushed and avoided, similar, perhaps, to the ignored abuse of children by Catholic priests. Sooner or later, the truth will be told, and for Rebecca, this ultimately meant coming forward in the press (forget anonymity in this type of situation) and in court to prevent further abuse to other women.

Before beginning her story, Rebecca felt it important to mention that professional counselors are supposed to adhere to a code of ethical and moral boundaries to assure those seeking help that their rights will be respected and that the counselor will act in a professional manner. There are several variations, but this condensed information is from the Center for the Prevention of Sexual and Domestic Violence in Seattle, Washington.

Sexual Abuse within the Ministerial Relationship happens when someone in a ministerial role (clergy, religious or lay) engages in sexual contact or sexualized behavior with a congregant, employee, student or counseling client in the ministerial relationship.

Sexual abuse can include *physical contact* from the person in the ministerial role, such as
- sexual touch and "accidental" touch of sexual areas of the body
- tickling and playful aggression that seem uncomfortable to you
- a prolonged hug when a brief hug is customary behavior
- kissing on the lips when a kiss on the cheek would be appropriate
- pressing up against your body when hugging
- an inappropriate gift from the professional such as lingerie
- sexual intercourse

Sexual abuse can also include *verbal behavior* initiated by a person in a min-

isterial role when such behavior sexualizes a relationship. Examples include:
- innuendo or sexual talk
- suggestive comments
- tales of the counselor's sexual exploits or experiences
- questions about the intimate details of your relationships
- looking for sympathy about his or her partner's sexual inadequacies
- inviting you to hot tub or swim naked, etc.

How do you know if your boundaries have been crossed?
- You feel uncomfortable and confused with the interaction even if you are initially flattered.
- You are receiving personal gifts from your minister or counselor.
- When you need the professional for counseling, you end up talking more about his or her problems than about yours
- The counselor is inviting you out for intimate, social occasions
- The minister or counselor touches you in a way that you find confusing, uncomfortable or upsetting
- The minister or counselor gives you theological rationale for questionable conduct, e.g. "God has brought us together."

Sexual contact within the ministerial relationship is a violation of professional ethics. There is a difference in power between a person in a ministerial role and a member of his or her congregation or a counselee. You cannot give *meaningful consent* to sexual contact since there is a difference in power between you.

You will seek counseling or support from your clergyman usually at times of stress or crisis in your life. During these times, you are vulnerable emotionally and can be taken advantage of by a minister who does not do what is best for you.

***

Rebecca's story is a classic example of boundary violations by a clergyman that began in her first year of sobriety. Her counselor had just allowed her to realize how she had been a victim for years of emotional incest. Physically and mentally drained, she broke down crying in an AA meeting in a small church. A well-meaning fellow AA took her to the pastor's office.

"I was hysterical," she said. "Right away, he calmed me down and was interested in my situation."

She pointed out that this clergyman had a reputation for helping alcoholics in the community and was also recognized by local law enforcement as a source of help for alcoholics.

"At the time I met him I was five months sober, very vulnerable and had just completed Step Three of the program. He said that, with my sponsor's permission, he'd take me back to the second step and that he would do the steps with me. Because the Big Book mentions using a clergyman for the Fifth Step, and because my sponsor thought so much of this person, she gave her permission. I was literally swept off my feet that this known clergyman would take an interest in me."

It wasn't until much later that she found out that many women with father or incest issues were also counseled by him with disastrous abuse results.

For the next year and a half, Rebecca met with him at times of her choosing. The door was always open to her, with no formal scheduled appointments, which she later found out was a boundary violation.

"No one else could see him at any time," she said. "At the time it made me feel special, which is what he wanted. In a year and a half we were at the Tenth Step and had discussed every aspect of my personal life. The problem was, again another boundary violation, that he began to discuss his personal life with me. He would disclose personal things about himself, convincing me that his marriage was ruined and that he was a victim, that his wife did not have the wonderful qualities I possessed. I was his hostage, HIS victim." she said, shaking her head as if to again rid herself of the emotional chains.

Through her women friends, Rebecca found out that the clergyman's wife (his fourth) was much younger than he, recovering from alcoholism, and that she had gone to his office for counseling after being raped by her father. He divorced his current, third wife and married her, his fourth wife, when she became pregnant with his child. Rebecca entered his office after their second child was born, supposedly his eighth child overall. But because he was a man of the cloth, no one publicly talked about his past or present involvement with women, and in reality, many recovering alcoholic men who knew him and heard his story continued to look up to him as a macho hero and victim.

He told her things in confidence that she later found out he told to everyone.

"He was very seductive, telling me I was the only one he could trust," she said. "Then there was inappropriate touching, insinuations, double-meanings, things said to confuse me under the guise of help."

When she confided in him about her feelings toward him, he told her not to worry, there was no reason not to trust him.

She said the progression of physical abuse was subtle, beginning with hugs at the end of each counseling session. They progressively got more intimate, and then, six weeks before he ultimately ended counseling, he appeared at her apartment uninvited.

"I let him in, probably because my father issues and codependence made me very vulnerable," she said. "It's really all about power – the power of the clerical collar, the position, a man with connections, someone looked up to in the judicial system. I had this powerful man paying all this attention to me."

Rebecca said she struggled early with feelings of affection for him, which she now knows is a very normal occurrence of transference, but professional counselors are trained to know this will occur and are expected to maintain boundaries to protect the person seeking help.

"The situation could have become fully sexual with him, but at the last minute I just couldn't do it," she said. "I truly believe that God intervened and protected me. In that moment I experienced total revulsion."

After five years of therapy she fully understands why. Counseling is a form of reparenting and clergy sexual abuse of the counseling relationship is incest.

It was then that he dropped her from counseling, accusing her of ruining his marriage.

"I was devastated," she said. "It's a miracle I didn't drink, because he had isolated me over the months from my women friends in AA. I still had my sponsor, but she was as confused as me because she, too, looked up to this supposedly respected man of the clergy who helped alcoholics recover. I still wanted to trust the God side of him because he became my higher power when I had no God coming into recovery. I know now that there are many trusted professionals who hide behind a degree or collar who are actually sexual predators and/or sociopaths. You'll find them wherever there are people in pain. Some people find it hard to believe that an adult can be abused the same as a child. They just don't get it."

She said once the church became aware of what the clergyman was doing, he was let go, defrocked, but with an ego beyond belief, the clergyman put his collar back on, started his own church and continued living life as if nothing happened.

"I just wasn't getting over what happened to me," she said, "and then he moved into the building next to my parents who were both Alzheimer's patients. When I realized I'd have to look at that slimy man every day or that he might approach and touch my invalid mother in her wheelchair I was galvanized into action. Other survivors of his abuse had begun coming to me, and I had this huge picture that included incest in his family and physical abuse of his wife. Twenty-seven women disclosed he had made inappropriate sexual advances during his counseling. He married two former counselees and another escaped out of state. As more and more women came forward, God led my determination to file a lawsuit, to put an end to his abuse and to expose the clergyman. Lawyers offered to take the case. I decided to let God work though them and let the process unfold. It did not take the direction I had hoped, because I wanted to get him personally. Instead, they went after the church that had continued supporting him despite allegations over the years."

After a seven-day trial, the church was found negligent in hiring and supervising him, and the jury found that Rebecca was sexually battered by him, that he intentionally inflicted emotional abuse on her. Although the suit was not against him personally, he had to testify.

"Basically, the jury didn't buy his story," she said. "I got tremendous validation through him testifying."

Until recently, the First Amendment protected the clergy. Rebecca was fortunate to live in a state where the supreme court decided clergy can't hide behind the separation of church and state, that licensed counselors weren't protected from felony charges.

"When I won the case women all over the United States cheered," she said., "but at first it was bittersweet because some one person on the jury didn't get it that an adult in counseling could be abused. I am at peace with it, though, because there are people who are simply incapable of comprehending that an adult can be abused. No amount of explaining will change that."

Her survivor friends keep reminding her of how a reporter described her as elegant and well-spoken.

"I exposed the perpetrator, I got validation and I maintained my dignity. That's an awesome outcome."

Years later, this clergyman is still practicing behind the

shield of his own church. Recently, a young woman new to AA was given his phone number for counseling. Her sponsor told her not to call. The young woman said, "but he's a minister, he's old, what's the danger?"

Rebecca shook her head.

"I still step forward, but I can't control him," she said. "The best thing is for women to become aware that not every professional IS professional."

Since winning the case, Rebecca has helped many women across the country who have suffered similar situations. She was on email with a woman in India about advocating for a woman survivor in California abused by a Buddhist priest.

"I thought this was incredible to be writing a woman in the Himalayas trying to help someone else across the world," she said. "We are all in this together, no matter where we are."

She met with another woman devastated by a Catholic priest in California. She has been on email for three years with a woman in a small farming town in Nebraska who was isolated and shunned after falling prey to her predator pastor.

"In recovery we become aware that our lives do serve a purpose, that the more we are aware and the healthier we become mentally, physically and emotionally, the more people we can serve," she said. "I feel we should bloom in place, give meaning to where we are and what we're doing. God has brought us through diversity and hurt in order to serve others. Many survivors lose their faith. I share the God I have been given in recovery."

***

For Angie, the issue for counseling was her marriage. While she and her husband had been to marriage counseling (and sex counseling) in early sobriety, it didn't work, not because of the counselors, but because both parties have to truly WANT the marriage to continue.

"Every time we seemed to progress and I felt comfortable with the process, my husband would decide he didn't want to continue," she said. They would go home, "half-baked" as they were, and wait for the cake to flop once again.

"When my pain and frustration became unbearable, I suggested marriage counseling once again at about five years sober. His reply was that he didn't want to go through all that pain again. I said, 'Okay, then I'll go by myself.' And I did."

A woman counselor had been recommended to Angie by her sponsor, so she made an appointment with her.

"She was in Al-Anon, was the oldest in a family of many siblings like myself, and seemed to grasp the situation on the initial interview. She also asked that I make a commitment of at least six months."

Angie agreed, and the journey began. Each weekly session uncovered more discomfort, doubt, fear and anger. She realized she had a lot of self-loathing in accepting the positions of care-giver, provider, defender and nurturer.

"I truly felt the brunt of responsibility not only in keeping the marriage and family together, but also the business that we had developed," she said. "I was overloaded, unloved, not appreciated and taken for granted. I was not only angry at my spouse, but myself. Through delicate surgery each week, we looked at the issues, found where I was at fault for allowing all this to happen, and worked on solutions."

Because the counseling was one-sided concerning the marriage, it became evident in the first few weeks that Angie was beating a dead horse.

"The marriage had been over for quite some time," she said. "I was just the last to know. By not wanting to go to counseling once again, my husband had, in effect, told me it was over. He just didn't have the courage to verbalize his feelings or to initiate divorce proceedings. I felt resentful that, once again, the burden was on me to do all the work. But I also knew it had to be done."

Her counselor pointed out that she would need a family car.

"My children had long outgrown my little sports car, although I still stuffed them into it when their father's car wasn't available," she laughed. "Letting go of that one item was a monumental step in my growth process. I sold it and succumbed to driving a four-door sedan style car with lots of room in the trunk."

That minor change was a major event in Angie's life. It represented "throwing in the towel" concerning the marriage. It gave her the strength to proceed to the next step.

"Because there were almost two years of separation before the divorce was final, I was able to look at my issues, stand back from them, and have the courage to make the necessary changes."

Then one day her counselor told Angie they wouldn't be seeing each other again, at least not as counselor/patient.

"She gave me the green light to go it alone in life, reassuring me that I could always seek help again if I ever needed it. Leaving her office that day I felt healthy, whole, lovable, talented, witty, wonderful," she said. "Finally, I felt 'there.'"

Block by block my imaginary wall began to crumble. I could see slivers of sun shining through the crumbling chinks. I let you see me, every minute detail, all those things the wall hid and protected. A gentle wind blew through the openings, clearing the settled dust. I shoved the debris away, wanting to help, to be free. But just as the wall took years to build, it was slow to dismantle. Instant freedom was not for this prisoner. Block by block, awareness by feeling, by thinking, by opening my heart, my very soul tore down my prison. Oh sunlight! Where have I been? Where am I going? I fear stumbling as I walk the road away from my wall, unaccustomed to going forward. But the light is so inviting, so strong. Where have I been?

Angie's writings 1989

***

Angie spoke of another incident involving professional counselors. Years ago she was invited to address a group of psychiatrists and psychologists on the opening of a new treatment center in the area. A 10-minute announcement soon turned into an hour-long confrontation as they questioned the nature of her disease.

"I found myself defending alcoholism and AA as the best treatment, as few of the 25 professionals in the room at the time considered it a disease. I finally asked for a show of hands on how many had ever attended an AA meeting to find out what it was all about," she said. "Only three raised their hands, the three who seemed to understand my position, nodding their heads as I spoke. I ultimately accused the others of catering to the disease by prescribing mood altering drugs, which meant they were more interested in profit than prevention."

She pointed out that giving drugs to an alcoholic or addict only feeds their disease.

"The alcoholic goes to a professional because she doesn't know where to turn," she said. "She trusts that the professional will be truthful. If the problem is alcoholism, then AA is the answer, along with treatment if necessary. If there are other problems such as depression or bipolar disorder, then these should be treated with the knowledge that the patient is also alcoholic. Counseling should enhance the AA program of recovery, not hinder it."

Times have changed in the past 15 years since this incident happened, but it's still important that those seeking help for alcoholism be aware that there are some professionals more interested in filling their calendar and/or prolonging recovery by prescribing drugs than referring someone to a free program.

"Perhaps they are not aware of what they are doing, but the qualified professional knows that Alcoholics Anonymous offers the best treatment for the disease of alcoholism," she said.

Suggestions for getting professional help

- ❀ This decision is usually made during difficult stress, but take the time to find out about the professional you choose.
- ❀ Try to find someone who specializes in your problem: addictions, sexual abuse, divorce, family, mental disorders, etc. Many professionals are skilled in related fields, with emphasis on one or another. Follow what your heart tells you, asking God to guide the way to the person who is supposed to help you.
- ❀ Get a referral from someone who has been to a particular therapist. Ask for a free consultation before agreeing to therapy. Don't hesitate to interview more than one. If you feel uncomfortable at all, interview another counselor until you're reasonably sure this is the person you want to hear your life history.
- ❀ Make sure boundaries are discussed at the beginning of counseling. You have a right to know what feelings may develop as a result of counseling so that you can be open and honest with your professional without fear of abuse.
- ❀ It's normal to develop strong feelings during counseling and it's important to discuss these with your therapist. It's a good idea for women to seek women counselors.
- ❀ Some AAs think you can get sober and healthy just through the program. Do not be bullied. Do what's best for you. The Big Book encourages outside professional help when needed.
- ❀ Be willing to make a long-term commitment. You didn't get this way overnight and it may take months,

maybe years, to deal with problems accumulated over a lifetime. A good counselor will get you there. Just peel off the layers one at a time. Sometimes you'll need a break...just know that it's long-term however the time frame unfolds. Everyone has different issues and situations.

Other Issues
National Tragedy – 9/11/01

I had no vision for including thoughts of a national tragedy in this book prior to September 11, 2001, but my first reaction after the initial shock of watching our symbols of commerce, democracy and freedom crumble was concern about alcoholics in New York, Washington, those close to passengers on the Pennsylvania flight who may have lost loved ones, and about those who would be in the midst of the chaos helping others. I remember saying a prayer that they not think the world was over and pick up a drink. I prayed that they would get to a meeting, call their sponsors, talk to one another. News, both happy and tragic, is always a reason for an alcoholic to drink..

In talking to Angie about the tragedy, she said taking a drink was the furthest thing from her mind that dreadful day as emergency workers waited to treat patients who perished without having a chance, as heroic firemen and policemen tirelessly tried to find anyone still alive.

"I felt paralyzed with the rest of my fellow Americans as we watched hour by hour the rescue and recovery efforts, joined together in our sorrow and the reality of the rubble," she said.

With tears again in her eyes, Angie expressed how she felt vulnerable, violated, angry, incensed. She felt resentment, hate and a desire to "get even."

"I felt grief, I felt relief that I was at a distance from the horror, then felt guilty because I felt relief," she said. "Every emotion surfaced. The overwhelming sadness that was shared by all was immeasurable."

During that time she spoke at an AA meeting.

"Before telling my story, I felt compelled to talk about the importance of voicing our feelings, of being human and allowing our emotions to unfold, about the emptiness, the fear, the incredible sadness. If we are to heal, we MUST feel."

When she was still drinking she was numb.

"Today I am aware, I can be fearful while knowing that God has a bigger plan. I can feel my own pain, but, more importantly, the pain of others," she said. "I can cry, I can talk to strangers and I can pray."

With the little things in life she has conditioned herself to ask "How important is it?" And so it is with the big things.

"This was an important, tragic, murderous, hateful event that brought a nation to its knees in prayer," she said. "Thank God as an alcoholic I had a place to turn with my pain, other women to talk to about my feelings, and a God of my understanding who opened my heart to pray for fellow alcoholic women faced with grievous loss in the tragedy, to ask God to help them."

Just as Alcoholics Anonymous is comprised of people of every race, religion, color and creed with the sole purpose of staying sober and helping one another, we watched our leaders of every party and persuasion come together with the sole purpose of preserving our freedom and helping one another – individual or nation.

This tragedy emphasized how important it is to live TODAY.

"We never know what will happen tomorrow," said Angie. "If we are right in our hearts and spirit today, if we stay sober and help another alcoholic, it doesn't matter what happens tomorrow. God will give us the strength, courage and ability to know what to do. We need only to pray for His will."

Just as alcohol brought Angie to her knees, 9/11/01 brought this great nation to its knees. The terrorists were "cunning, baffling, and powerful," holding us hostage just as alcohol once held Angie. With God and faith and "doing the right thing," their evil hold on the world will be released.

In the days and weeks that followed Angie found it difficult to shake an incredible sadness...for her country, for the poor helpless, persecuted women and children of Afghanistan.

"I found myself praying more than usual, knowing that, as always, God was the answer when nothing else made sense."

Using the Internet

When Angie got sober the Internet didn't exist, but today it is another useful tool for women who want to get and stay sober. There are meetings online, there are chat rooms that provide instant "conscious contact" and women who have gone through similar difficulties who offer their help online. As in meetings, not everyone you encounter online will have quality sobriety. It's important to use the Internet only as a supplement to "real" meetings and a sponsor you can look in the eye.

Any alcoholic woman who is unable to get to meetings because of health problems or lack of transportation can search for an online home group to have contact with good sobriety. There are many women with years in the program who are now shut-ins relying on the Internet for meetings. Angie joked that the AA program founders probably never dreamed that "going to any length" would someday include using a computer!

Finding meetings online is easy. Just search for "AA meetings online" and it will give several Web sites to visit, including http://www.stayingcyber.org and http://www.aaonline.net for AOL users. Alcoholics Anonymous has a home page with general information as well as links to literature, newsletters, general service offices worldwide, press releases and other useful topics: http://www.alcoholics-anonymous.org. There is also a link to the organization's monthly magazine *AA Grapevine*, a "meeting in print" at http://www.aagrapevine.org.

Sometimes we find ourselves in a situation where there is no one in our local recovery community who has experienced the particular problem we face, or we may have a delicate situation involving someone in the clergy, the professional community or in the public eye. The Internet can be a valuable resource for comfort and direction for that situation.

For abuse by professional clergy or counselor, which can be a sensitive topic to discuss with someone in the local community, Rebecca highly recommends visiting http://www.advocateweb.com as a source of information and hope that includes legal, moral, health care and ethical issues, as well as sources for mental and spiritual help.

News Media

Many recovering alcoholics were incensed over a television segment on *20/20* that expounded on how AA is not all that successful and that possibly alcoholism is not a disease. A program like this only lets the person in denial continue the progression of drinking. Whether or not it is a "disease" it is a predictable killer for all those who have become addicted. Statistics state that approximately 80 percent of the population can drink successfully. These people may have casual drinks and drunks to celebrate occasions, but their personalities basically remain the same. They know the consequences of their actions and are free to make choices to either stop drinking or do it again with the same consequence. They are not addicted to alcohol.

But for the alcoholic, loss of control is totally predictable, not all the time, but with the number of problems increasing in direct proportion to consumption. The program talked about a British woman who allows herself "points" per week for drinking. She obviously is fighting control over alcohol. Why be so hung up on what you are allowing yourself when those thoughts and energies could be put into recovery?

So what if arresting the disease means abstinence? If a person were told that carrots caused his cancer and that if he stopped eating carrots the cancer would go away, it's a no-brainer what his decision would be.

But alcohol is different. It's cunning, baffling and powerful, just like the "Big Book" says in Chapter 5 of How it Works. It tells you it's not a disease, that it's everyone else's fault, and that you're really okay.

How *20/20* could cite all the statistics of the effects of alcohol in our prisons, mental institutions and hospitals, to say nothing of the number of deaths due to homicide, vehicle accidents and overdoses each year, and not see a connection with a very serious problem (disease or not) makes no sense.

Alcohol ruins lives, families and innocent bystanders. To work on a "cure" is ludicrous, to bash AA is senseless. It works for those willing to believe in a Power greater than themselves. No rules, no regulations, no one keeping score. It's a simple program of honesty enlisting the help of a spiritual nature. It's true that possibly only one in 35 who come to AA "makes it." It's not an easy program to grasp, but it sure is simple once the fog clears, the alcohol drains out of the system and health – mental, spiritual and physical – returns.

It is no doubt that many alcoholics on the verge of recovery were set back by this television program based on information from people who simply didn't want to give up alcohol. It's hard enough staying sober even when you KNOW the truth about the disease.

An interesting footnote to this story: It was later reported that the woman who allowed herself "points" for drinking ended up with points of another nature. She was picked up for driving under the influence, unable to control what we know is her disease.

***

Since the time Angie got sober, much has changed in terms of public information about alcoholism and addiction. There are now public service messages, commercials about addiction and getting help, and many television shows portray addiction and recovery as part of everyday life. We have seen celebrities sent off to treatment, many more than one time. We've seen compassion and understanding replace judgement and disgust. We've watched movies tell our own story, and we have witnessed a tremendous, encouraging change. We can go to the Internet and find out everything there is to know about alcoholism and recovery.

"Twenty years ago I would have been uncomfortable admitting to or talking about my alcoholism," said Angie. "Today I am proud to be among the growing population of those in recovery. People readily ask questions today that would have been taboo years ago. Alcoholism has been one of the major killers, a known fatal disease for years, but only recently has it been properly categorized and recognized."

Because addiction affects virtually every family in some way, more people are getting help through treatment and/or Alcoholics Anonymous. Whole families are getting help with Al-Anon. The horrible shame once attached to the alcoholic family member (Uncle So-and-So the town drunk) is met with more acceptance and knowledge of the illness. This doesn't mean the alcoholic gets help or is even tolerated by the family, but because there has been so much information on alcoholism and addiction the family can no longer be totally ignorant of the disease or treatment. If the alcoholic does not receive help, it's by choice.

This has been particularly helpful for women alcoholics, because if it's portrayed on television and in the movies, it must be okay to talk about it, and even fashionable to go for treatment. For years it was considered mainly a man's problem. He took pride in being able to hold his own at the local bar. If a woman family member drank she was kept at home and no one talked about her "situation." Today we know that alcoholism plays no favorites. Men, women, children, rich or poor, illiterate or Ph.D., black or white, Christian, Muslim, Jew or atheist – it doesn't matter.

Just as heart disease kills people throughout the world, so too does alcoholism. What's interesting is that the "cure" is so simple. It doesn't require heart transplants or daily insulin shots, it doesn't require constant monitoring of vital functions. The alcoholic merely has to stop drinking to begin recovery from alcoholism.

Simple, yet difficult.

Simple, yet successful.

Simple, yet the disease will keep denying itself, whispering to the committee in the head of its host to pay it no mind, to just have another drink.

Simple, if we ask for God's help.

I can't, He can, I think I'll let Him.

About the Author

Martha (Marty) Crikelair Wohlford is a professional writer who brings a wealth of knowledge and experience to her work. She has sailed all her life, is a private pilot, diver, photographer, musician, and graphic artist.

She is a graduate of St. Mary's College, Notre Dame, Ind., where she majored in English Literature and Creative Writing. Her career began as a feature writer/editor for several newspapers and magazines. She established her own public relations firm in the early 1970s, and her combination of photography, writing and graphics skills have resulted in numerous brochures, catalogs, ads, websites and image pieces for a variety of clients.

She has also written *Drumbeat No Lie*, a novel of murder, intrigue and romance that takes place in the Bahamas, and two children's books: *Little Star's Big Day*, a Christmas story, and *Splash, the Staniel Cay Cat*.

Marty spends most of her time at her home in Staniel Cay, Exumas, Bahamas, where she continues to write , enjoy life, and nourish her spirit.

Internet: www.mwpr.com
email:marty@mwpr.com

Drumbeat No Lie
A novel by Martha Crikelair Wohlford

Drumbeat No Lie is a fictional caper that involves drug smugglers operting on a laid-back, pristine little island many years ago somewhere in the Bahamas. Where pirates and rumrunners once plied the waters under sail, the drug cartels now use speedboats and helicopters – and the cargo is not pludered gold ande booze, but pot and cocaine.

Woody Cameron sets up operations at an abandoned island resort that he has purchased, recruiting help among the riffraff eager to make a big score and the free spirits hoping to bankroll an island-hopping cruise, courtesy of the drug trade. Pete Mathews, proprietor of the Sandy Cay Club on a neighboring island, keeps a watchful and disgusted eye on Cameron and the comings and goings of his henchmen.

This is a story of intrigue, drug busts, murder, and romance, with its share of humorous, rock-happy characters. Anyone who has visited the Bahamas or or dreamed of visiting the Caribbean will be caught up in the story.

Comments:

"Very good writing, very snappy and crisp. I find it not only inviting but compelling and really like all the visual pictures you paint along the way. You're especially good at creating tactile characters. They're so real, as if the reader can touch them, feel them, embrace them, They are certainly easy to relate to." Harry Hilson • Fine Art, Inc.

"I don't want it to end." June • Bahamas

"I feel like I know all your characters. I find myself talking to people about them as though they exist. Write more books!" Mary S. • Haverton, PA

"I read your book and loved it. How clever and talented you are." Judith J. • South Bend, IN

Paperback: ISBN: 978-0-9787981-1-6

www.ingramcontent.com/pod-product-compliance
Lightning Source LLC
Chambersburg PA
CBHW022359040426
42450CB00005B/250